Radiation Health and Safety Exam Practice Questions

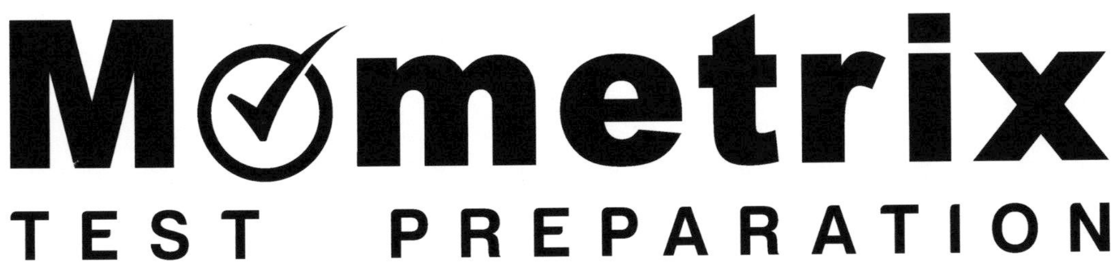

Dear Future Exam Success Story

First of all, **THANK YOU** for purchasing Mometrix study materials!

Second, congratulations! You are one of the few determined test-takers who are committed to doing whatever it takes to excel on your exam. **You have come to the right place.** We developed these practice tests with one goal in mind: to deliver you the best possible approximation of the questions you will see on test day.

Standardized testing is one of the biggest obstacles on your road to success, which only increases the importance of doing well in the high-pressure, high-stakes environment of test day. Your results on this test could have a significant impact on your future, and these practice tests will give you the repetitions you need to build your familiarity and confidence with the test content and format to help you achieve your full potential on test day.

Your success is our success

We would love to hear from you! If you would like to share the story of your exam success or if you have any questions or comments in regard to our products, please contact us at **800-673-8175** or **support@mometrix.com**.

Thanks again for your business and we wish you continued success!

Sincerely,
The Mometrix Test Preparation Team

Written and edited by the Mometrix Exam Secrets Test Prep Team
Printed in the United States of America

TABLE OF CONTENTS

RHS Practice Test #1

1. Which of the following factors causes collimator cutoff?

a. The central ray was not directed at center of the image receptor.
b. There was excessive vertical angle.
c. The plane of the image receptor was not flat.
d. There was too much exposure.

2. The primary disadvantage of the bisecting technique when contrasted with the paralleling technique is:

a. Longer exposure time.
b. Dimensional distortion of the teeth.
c. Requirement of an image receptor holder.
d. Greater magnification.

3. What is the name of the device used to monitor employees for radiation exposure?

a. Radiographometer
b. Oximeter
c. Holter monitor
d. Dosimeter

4. The dental radiographer places the digital sensor in the patient's mouth and exposes it to radiation, hearing the notification that radiation was emitted. No image appears on the computer screen. What is the cause of this error?

a. The sensor was placed in the mouth backward; therefore, the active part of the sensor was not facing the position-indicating device (PID).
b. The PID was missing a portion of the digital sensor.
c. The dental radiographer used too much vertical angle resulting in foreshortening and missing the structure being radiographed.
d. The milliamperage setting was set too low, resulting in the image not being visible to the dental team.

5. Which one of the following is a feature of digital imaging that allows the dental assistant to flip the image so that the dark areas will appear light and the light areas will appear dark?

a. Charged coupling
b. Digital subtraction
c. Pixel reversal
d. Storage phosphor imaging

6. According to the American Academy of Oral and Maxillofacial Radiology, how often should an x-ray machine be tested?

a. Every 6 months
b. Annually
c. Biannually
d. Every 3 years

7. Which one of the following is a clinical contact surface that is commonly contaminated during dental imaging?

a. Radiographic machine control panel
b. Operatory sink
c. Dental chair foot pedal
d. The viewing window that connects the dental radiographer to the patient

8. In reference to the density of a dental image, nonpathological conditions appearing as distinctive black areas can be identified as:

a. composite restorations.
b. bone.
c. amalgam fillings.
d. air spaces.

9. Which of the following statements is TRUE?

a. Scattered radiation affects the patient and the radiographer.
b. Scattered radiation is not dangerous.
c. Scattered radiation is absorbed by the patient's skin.
d. Scattered radiation is useful in the production of the latent image.

10. Which one of the following is accurate when describing how an all-porcelain bridge or crown will appear on a dental image?

a. The crown or bridge will appear as a white or radiopaque area that covers the entire tooth but allows for some see-through areas.
b. The crown or bridge will always appear dark or radiolucent.
c. The crown or bridge will appear on the front teeth only and will appear completely white or radiopaque.
d. The crown or bridge will appear as white or radiopaque restorations and will always have a slight outline on the outside of the restoration where the porcelain comes away from the underlying surface.

11. When exposing dental radiographs, which of the following position indicating devices (PIDs) will produce the least amount of magnification?

a. 8 inch.
b. 12 inch.
c. 16 inch.
d. 20 inch.

12. When using digital wired sensors, which one of the following infection control procedures is accurate?

a. Place the wired sensor into the patient's oral cavity, capture the image, remove the sensor from the oral cavity, place the sensor in the ultrasonic machine, and disinfect the sensor.
b. Place the wired sensor into the barrier, place it into the patient's oral cavity, remove the sensor from the oral cavity, disinfect the sensor, and place the sensor in the dry heat sterilizer.
c. Place the wired sensor into the barrier, place this into the patient's oral cavity, remove the barrier with the sensor from the oral cavity, remove the sensor from the barrier, and disinfect the sensor.
d. Place the wired sensor into the patient's oral cavity, capture the image, remove the sensor from the oral cavity, disinfect the sensor, and place the sensor into the autoclave for sterilization.

13. Which one of the following accurately reflects the standard of care when working with patients who have special needs?

a. When working with a patient with visual impairment, quietly enter and exit the room while providing dental treatment so as not to startle the patient.
b. When working with a patient with hearing impairment, per statute, they must always have an interpreter present for dental care.
c. Avoid asking patients questions about their disability that are not related to the care they will receive at the dental office.
d. For patients who have a strong gag reflux, increase the tactile stimuli, and ask the patient to briefly hold their breath as you place the digital receptor.

14. What is the correct method for disinfecting phosphor storage plates (PSPs)?

a. The dental radiographer removes the PSP from the patient's mouth with gloved hands, places it in the PSP scanner, retrieves it from the PSP scanner, removes the barrier, and wipes it with the appropriate disinfectant.
b. The dental radiographer removes the PSP from the patient's mouth with gloved hands, removes the barrier, wipes the PSP with the appropriate disinfectant, and places it in the PSP scanner.
c. The patient removes the PSP from the oral cavity, removes the barrier, and transfers the PSP to the dental radiographer, who then wipes it with the appropriate disinfectant and places it in the PSP scanner.
d. The patient or the dental radiographer removes the PSP from the oral cavity, removes the barrier, places the PSP into the PSP scanner, retrieves it from the PSP scanner, and then wipes it with the appropriate disinfectant.

15. What is the setting that controls the number of electrons that are produced within the dental tubehead?

a. Kilovoltage peak
b. Thermionic emission
c. Milliamperage selector
d. Kinetic energy

16. Which of the following is correct when mounting and labeling digital images?

a. Digital images may be moved around the screen to allow for proper mount placement.
b. It is common practice to print out a copy of digital images, cut them out, and place them into a clear plastic mount when requested by a dental office.
c. Each digital recording should be saved with a minimum of the patient's last name and date of birth.
d. When exposing digital images, there is only one size mount that is available in the digital imaging software on the screen.

17. When considering collimation selection, what type of collimator produces the least amount of excess radiation to a patient?

a. Rectangular.
b. Cone shaped.
c. Circular.
d. They all have the same effects on the patient; it is the length that makes the difference.

18. Which one of the following anatomical structures will be found in the maxillary molar periapical image?

a. Lingual foramen
b. Median palatine suture
c. Hamulus
d. Mental ridge

19. Identify the unit of time used to measure how long x-rays are emitted from the dental tubehead:

a. Amperes.
b. Milliamperes.
c. Volts.
d. Impulses.

20. Which type of radiation results from the interaction of the primary beam with matter?

a. Background.
b. Primary.
c. Secondary.
d. Stray.

21. Infection prevention practices that must be followed during dental imaging include all of the following EXCEPT:

a. The use of protective PPE
b. Avoiding cross contamination of imaging devices
c. Properly disposing of waste materials
d. Avoiding the use of disposable items

22. Which one of the following is a required step to complete before exposing a patient to dental images?

a. Remove the barrier from the sensor and disinfect the sensor.
b. If using phosphor storage plates (PSPs), remove the barrier and wipe down the PSPs.
c. Wipe down the patient apron.
d. Remove sterilized items from their packaging, and assemble any receptor-holding devices.

23. Which of the following structures will be visible on a mandibular periapical??

a. Lingual foramen
b. Incisive foramen
c. Coronoid process
d. Median palatine suture

24. When viewing dental radiographs, which anatomical landmark can be of assistance in identifying the maxillary central periapical image?

a. The coronoid process.
b. The mental ridge.
c. The median palatine suture.
d. The external oblique.

25. When finished with all radiographic exposures, the patient apron can be removed aseptically from the patient in all of the following ways EXCEPT:

a. by removing the apron with contaminated gloves.
b. by removing the apron with the use of overgloves.
c. by removing the apron after the removal of contaminated gloves, followed by handwashing.
d. by removing the apron barehanded.

26. Which of the following is a type of indirect digital imaging used in dentistry?

a. Wired digital sensor.
b. Storage phosphor imaging.
c. A panoramic digital image.
d. Charge-coupled sensor.

27. What size of position-indicating device (PID) is more effective in reducing patient exposure?

a. 5 inch.
b. 8 inch.
c. 16 inch.
d. 14 inch.

28. Which of the following statements is TRUE regarding radiation protection to the dental radiographer?

a. The dental radiographer is able to stand in the line of the direct beam once.
b. The dental radiographer should stand six feet or closer to the x-ray unit during exposure.
c. If a lead barrier is not available for the dental radiographer to stand behind, they should stand at a right angle to the beam.
d. If a lead barrier is not available for the dental radiographer to stand behind, they should not stand at a right angle to the beam.

29. The bisecting angle technique:

a. must be used with only a short position-indicating device (PID).
b. must be used with only a long PID.
c. must be used with only an eight-inch PID.
d. can be used with any length PID.

30. Which one of the following is an anatomical structure that will be visible in a maxillary periapical image?

a. Mental foramen
b. Genial tubercle
c. Mastoid process
d. Median palatine suture

31. Which one of the following is correct when it comes to infection control management for the dental imaging team?

a. The team must develop an optional postexposure management plan.
b. The dentist can serve as the professional in charge of evaluating any potential exposures.
c. The team must identify the procedures that pose risks to the dental team and outline how they should be carried out.
d. It should be mandated that reports of exposure within the dental office are not shared with outside agencies or parties, decreasing the risk of negative publicity for the dental radiographer and the office.

32. Which of the following statements is correct?

a. The longer the wavelength of the x-ray, the greater is its energy.
b. The shorter the wavelength of the x-ray, the lesser is its energy.
c. The shorter the wavelength of the x-ray, the greater is its energy.
d. The absence of the wavelength of the x-ray, the greater is its energy.

33. Distortion and overlapping of dental anatomy as seen on a panoramic image are caused by:

a. structures being captured within the focal trough.
b. structures being captured outside the focal trough.
c. structures being captured within the Curve of Spee.
d. structures being captured outside the Curve of Spee.

34. In what part of the x-ray machine are the x-rays produced?

a. X-ray tube
b. Tubehead
c. Control panel
d. Transformer

35. A standard full-mouth series of dental radiographs taken in general dentistry includes:

a. 14 periapicals, and 4 bitewings
b. 10 periapicals, and 8 bitewings
c. 14 periapicals,6 bitewings and a panoramic
d. 8 periapical views and 4 bitewings

36. Which one of the following statements is correct regarding the characteristics of x-rays used in dentistry?

a. The x-rays used in dentistry are low-frequency waves.
b. The x-rays used in dentistry are not considered ionizing radiation.
c. The x-rays used in dentistry have short wavelengths.
d. The x-rays used in dentistry do not have enough energy to cause tissue damage.

37. When the dentist needs to have a detailed view of the ramus area due to a suspected condylar neck fracture, which projection will they request from the dental assistant?

a. Temporomandibular joint projection.
b. Submentovertex projection.
c. Reverse Towne projection.
d. Waters projection.

38. During what stage of pregnancy is the fetus most sensitive to the effects of radiation exposure?

a. Weeks 2-15
b. Weeks 16-25
c. Weeks 26 and beyond
d. Sensitivity is uniform across the entire pregnancy.

39. Which one of the following is found on the mandibular central periapical image?

a. Lingual foramen
b. Mental foramen
c. Mandibular foramen
d. Incisive foramen

40. When exposing periapical and bitewing images, which error will result if the central ray is not aimed at the center of the receptor?

a. Overlapping
b. Ghost imaging
c. Cone cutting
d. Elongation

41. How would the dental team refer to a dental image that has few shades of gray?

a. An image with high contrast
b. An image with low contrast
c. An image with high density
d. An image with low density

42. Identify the kilovolt or kV setting that produces the greatest contrast among images on a radiograph:

a. 65 kV.
b. 75 kV.
c. 80 kV.
d. 90 kV.

43. Which of the following is used to control the penetrating power of the x-ray beam?

a. The milliamp selector.
b. The tubehead.
c. The kilovolt peak selector.
d. The tungsten filament.

44. Which of the following should be done to correct foreshortening?

a. Increase vertical angle.
b. Increase horizontal angle.
c. Decrease horizontal angle.
d. Decrease vertical angle.

45. Identify the part of the x-ray tube where the electrons turn into actual x-rays:

a. At the positively charged anode.
b. At the positively charged cathode.
c. At the negatively charged anode.
d. At the negatively charged cathode.

46. Which type of dental decay is not often viewable on a dental image?

a. Root surface
b. Interproximal
c. Incipient
d. Recurrent

47. What is a type of resorption viewable on a dental image that causes the root tips to become shortened due to known or unknown pressure?

a. Internal
b. Idiopathic
c. External
d. Physiologic

48. The dental assistant is exposing a full mouth series on an adult with a very narrow maxillary arch. What size image receptor should the dental auxiliary choose to allow for the best view of the maxillary anterior teeth?

a. Size 0.
b. Size 1.
c. Size 2.
d. Size 3.

49. A dental assistant experiences an occupational exposure. A patient's blood has splashed into the employee's eye. Which of the following is an appropriate next step to take?

a. Immediately draw blood from the patient in order to get it tested for HIV and HBV
b. Require the employee to have their own blood tested immediately for HIV and HBV
c. Document the incident, including the source individual, the employee, route of exposure, and how it happened
d. Check the patient's chart and determine if risk factors are present to warrant further testing for the employee

50. The type of radiograph that would show the whole tooth including the crown, roots, and jawline is called:

a. Bitewing
b. Periapical
c. Occlusal
d. Tomogram

51. What is the term used to describe the overall darkness of an image?

a. Contrast.
b. Density.
c. Overexposure.
d. Intensity.

52. Having the minimum object-image receptor distance is so important to eliminate:

a. tooth enlargement.
b. tooth shrinkage.
c. collimator cutoff.
d. cutoff of required structures.

53. Which one of the following is used to describe the process during which most, but not all, microbes are killed or removed from an item or surface?

a. Sterilization
b. Disinfection
c. Asepsis
d. Precleaning

54. Which one of the following statements regarding dental records and imaging is correct?

a. The dental team should store patient dental records for 5 years following the last dental visit.
b. It is acceptable to request that a patient transfer to a different dental practice if he or she will not allow the current dental team to capture dental images.
c. Patients can request only the financial aspects of their dental radiology records.
d. It is standard and acceptable practice for dental offices to capture images for every new patient.

55. Which one of the following is an example of something that is used with indirect digital imaging?

a. Phosphor storage plates
b. Gendex sensor
c. Processing chemicals
d. Analog imaging

56. Which one of the following is a required step for the dental radiographer to take in order to prevent disease transmission in the dental office?

a. Remove all PPE before leaving the dental operatory after dental imaging including eyewear, mask, gloves, and gowns/jackets.
b. Avoid hand washing if gloves were appropriately placed and remained intact during dental imaging.
c. Have the patient stay seated in the room for 10 minutes following the completion of dental imaging to allow the aerosols created by the procedure to settle from the air.
d. When a patient with a known infectious disease has dental images captured, the room, along with beam alignment devices and digital sensors, must receive double disinfection to prevent the spread of the infectious disease to other patients who will be in the room later.

57. Which one of the following is correct regarding the cleaning process for an extension cone paralleling device?

a. Proper processing includes precleaning and disinfection with a semicritical disinfectant.
b. Immersion sterilant is an acceptable option for sterilizing heat-stable beam alignment devices.
c. Disinfecting in ortho-phthalaldehyde (a high-level disinfectant) for 12 minutes is an acceptable processing technique for beam alignment devices.
d. Beam alignment devices are semicritical instruments and must be sterilized by heat if they are heat stable.

58. How will an intruded tooth appear on a dental image?

a. The intruded tooth will appear slightly out of the tooth socket.
b. The intruded tooth will appear slightly further into the tooth socket.
c. The intruded tooth will be removed from the socket.
d. The intruded tooth will appear with a small, circular dark area in its center.

59. Which of the following is FALSE regarding handwashing?

a. Alcohol-based hand gel can be used in place of soap and water on hands that are visibly dirty
b. Fingertips, thumbs, and between the fingers are 3 areas that are frequently not cleaned thoroughly with handwashing
c. Alcohol-based hand gel or foam should have a concentration of 60-95% alcohol
d. Cool water should be used to rinse hands after washing because it helps to close the pores in the skin

60. Which of the following choices describes a dental image with high contrast?

a. An image with many shades of gray
b. An overall a light image
c. An overall a dark image
d. An image with a few shades of gray

61. Which of the following is the required diameter of a collimated x-ray beam when it strikes the patient's face?

a. 2.75 inches.
b. 3.25 inches.
c. 3.50 inches.
d. 4.00 inches.

62. How is the *maximum accumulated lifetime dose* for healthcare workers calculated?

a. (*N*-18) x 5 rem/year
b. (*N*-10) x 5 rem/year
c. (*N*-18) x 10 rem/year
d. (*N*-10) x 10 rem/year

63. A patient is moving and asks for the most recent dental radiographs for their new dentist. Which of the following is NOT the preferred procedure for fulfilling this request?

a. Obtain the original images from the patient's record and give them to the patient to take to the new dentist
b. Prepare a copy of the images and allow the patient to take these to the dentist
c. Obtain contact information from the patient and mail to the new dentist
d. Obtain an email address for the new dentist and send the digital images electronically

64. Chronic radiation exposure to the lens of the eye may result in:

a. Astigmatism
b. Strabismus
c. Cataracts
d. Glaucoma

65. Which one of the following restorations is commonly used in children and will appear as slightly translucent on a dental image?

a. Composite filling
b. Gold crown
c. Stainless steel crown
d. Amalgam filling

66. Which one of the following is an example of a noncritical instrument or item used in dental imaging?

a. Bone chisel
b. Mouth mirror
c. Lead apron
d. Explorer

67. Which one the of the following is part of infection prevention in dental imaging?

a. The use of universal precautions
b. The use of additional infection control precautions for patients with bloodborne infectious diseases
c. The use of infection prevention practices before, during, and after dental imaging
d. The use of a minimizing beam alignment device

68. What causes overlap to been seen on a bitewing radiograph?

a. Incorrect vertical angulation of the position-indicating device (PID).
b. Incorrect alignment of the receptor in the area of the teeth being radiographed.
c. Incorrect kilovolt peak and milliamp settings.
d. Incorrect horizontal angulation of the PID.

69. Which organization determines the maximum permissible dose a healthcare provider can receive?

a. The National Council on Radiation Protection and Measurement.
b. OSHA.
c. FDA.
d. ADA.

70. When the Frankfort plane is positioned too high during the positioning of a patient for a panoramic image, the following result will occur:

a. a smile line curved upward.
b. a smile line curved downward.
c. the absence of a smile line.
d. a cone-shaped radiopacity that obscures the mandible.

71. When a patient presents with lingual tori, which of the following steps should the dental auxiliary take?

a. The patient will require a panoramic image due to the tori.
b. The image receptor should be placed on the torus and exposed.
c. The patient should be referred for surgical tori reduction before images are taken.
d. The image receptor must be placed on the far side of the torus.

72. Which of the following describes the use of an aluminum filter in a dental tubehead?

a. A filter reduces the size and shape of the beam.
b. A filter removes low-energy x-ray beams.
c. A filter removes the dose of radiation to the thyroid gland.
d. A filter decreases the mean energy of the beam.

73. All of the following would appear radiopaque on a periapical image EXCEPT:

a. a metal restoration.
b. dense cortical bone.
c. a sinus cavity.
d. maxillary tuberosity.

74. During x-ray production, the purpose of the step-down transformer is to:

a. decrease the voltage from 110 or 220 volts to 3 to 5 volts.
b. increase the voltage from 110 or 220 volts to 3 to 5 volts.
c. increase the voltage from 3 to 5 volts to 110 to 220 volts.
d. stop 110 or 220 volts from becoming 3 to 5 volts.

75. Which one of the following disinfectants has the ability to kill tuberculosis?

a. Enzymatic disinfectants
b. Intermediate-level disinfectants
c. Antiseptic disinfectants
d. Aseptic disinfectants

76. The Frankfurt plane is:

a. the top of ear lobe to top of eye socket.
b. the bottom of ear lobe to bottom of eye socket.
c. the bottom of ear cartilage to top of eye socket.
d. the opening of ear canal to bottom of eye socket.

77. Choose which of the following statements is FALSE:

a. Primary and secondary radiation are created when exposing a dental image.
b. Secondary radiation is not useful when exposing a dental image.
c. Primary radiation is created when the secondary radiation interacts with matter.
d. Secondary radiation can cause a fogging effect on dental radiographs.

78. Which one of the following actions is NOT appropriate when a dental radiographer receives a puncture through the skin or a splash to the eyes?

a. Wash the skin puncture area with soap and water, or flush the eyes with water.
b. Squeeze the punctured area to try to remove some of the microbes before applying antiseptics to the area.
c. Allow staff to provide first aid if applicable based on the injury severity.
d. Report the injury to the office infection control coordinator for further follow-up.

79. Which of the following causes overlapping?

a. Inadequate vertical angle.
b. Poor sagittal plane orientation.
c. Central ray not perpendicular to the teeth being exposed.
d. Patient movement.

80. Which one of the following can be visible on any dental image and will form a circular area near the tip of the tooth?

a. Periapical abscess
b. Apical foramen
c. Nasal cavity
d. Inferior nasal concha

Answer Key and Explanations for Test #1

1. A: Collimator cutoff, commonly referred to as cone cutting, occurs when the central ray was not directed at the center of the image receptor. This causes radiation to miss parts of the image receptor, resulting in a circular radiopaque area on the image receptor where dental structures should be. The dental auxiliary must always ensure they are covering their image receptor with the position indicator device prior to exposure to prevent this error.

2. B: The primary disadvantage of the bisecting technique is the dimensional distortion that may occur in the images that are taken using this technique. This is due to how the angulations are determined and how the central ray is aimed at an imaginary bisecting line that has been created by the angles of the image receptor and the long axis of the tooth. The paralleling technique should be used whenever possible due to the accuracy of the resulting images.

3. D: Occupational exposure to radiation should be kept at a minimum. Safety guidelines must be in place to help with this task. Radiation can be obtained from the primary source, leakage radiation, and scatter radiation. There are 3 types of monitoring devices available for employee use. A dosimeter measures the amount of radiation exposure. These are available as a pen style that can be worn in the pocket. A radiation monitoring badge can also be used and should be worn at all times while at work. After the end of monitoring period, the pen is sent to be processed to calculate the amount of radiation exposure. The third type is called a thermoluminescent dosimeter (TLD). X-ray equipment should be regularly serviced and monitored for leakage. Dental assistants must also take precautions while taking radiographs, such as avoiding the direct primary beam or standing behind the lead barrier, such as the appropriate wall.

4. A: When the dental assistant exposes an image, the x-ray machine will emit an audible sound indicating that x-rays have been produced and have been emitted from the tubehead. If that sound is heard but the computer screen does not receive an image, this indicates that the digital sensor was placed in the mouth backward so that the active part of the sensor was not placed toward the source of radiation. Therefore, the pixels were not energized by the radiation and no image was recorded. The dental assistant must correct this by ensuring that the active part of the sensor is facing the dental tubehead. If the PID is positioned over a portion of the sensor, there will be a partial image. If the dental assistant is using too much vertical angle, there will be a visible image that will have distortion or foreshortening in it. If the milliamperage setting is too low, the image that will result will be very light in color.

5. B: Digital subtraction is a viewing option found in dental software. It is when the dental radiographer can view the dark areas as light areas and the light areas as dark areas. This feature can be used when there is an area of question and the dental team needs a different view of the structure.

6. B: X-ray machines should be calibrated on a regular basis. There are both state and federal regulations in place regarding this issue. According to the American Academy of Oral and Maxillofacial Radiology, dental x-ray machines should be formally tested annually to ensure safety. The tests that should be done include x-ray output, kilovoltage calibration, milliamperage readings, timer accuracy, adequacy of collimation, alignment of the beam, and stability of the tubehead. Annual testing of these components will help to prevent malfunctioning of the x-ray machine. Results of this testing must be appropriately documented. It is important to store the extension arm in the closed position to help preserve the function of the tubehead. If left open all the time, the weight of the tubehead would likely cause the extension arm to weaken and cause radiation leakage.

7. A: A clinical contact surface is a type of environmental surface that is commonly contaminated during dental imaging and other dental procedures. Clinical contact surfaces must be precleaned and disinfected between each patient by using the appropriate disinfectant that will kill the types of microbes that are most commonly present on these types of surfaces in order to prevent cross contamination.

8. D: In reference to the density of a dental image, nonpathological conditions appearing as distinctive black areas can be identified as air spaces. This distinctive blackened area indicates that the x-ray beam was not obstructed by anything in its path during exposure. Exposure to bone will be indicated on the processed radiograph as white areas but with subtle porosities because the x-ray beam is unable to completely penetrate the bone due to its thickness and/or density. Amalgam fillings will appear completely opaque and white in color, without any opacity.

9. A: The true statement is as follows: "Scattered radiation affects the patient and the radiographer." This statement is true because it is unknown where the scattered radiation will be deflected to. Scattered radiation is not absorbed by the patient's skin because the skin acts as the matter in which the scattered radiation is deflected from.

10. A: When viewing all-porcelain bridges and/or crowns on a dental image, they will appear white but will allow for some see-through areas. This type of material is strong, but it does allow for some of the beam to pass through during the process of taking images. These beams then react with the digital parts of the sensor, allowing for the slightly see-through areas of the image. This is how this type of crown can be distinguished from gold crowns, stainless steel crowns, and porcelain fused to metal crowns.

11. C: The 16-inch position indicating device or PID will produce the least amount of image magnification on a dental radiograph. A maximum target to receptor distance is produced when a 16-inch PID is used. This, along with a minimum object-receptor distance, will give the dental radiographer the radiograph with the least amount of distortion and magnification.

12. C: The correct infection control procedure to follow when using direct digital imaging or imaging with a wired sensor is to place the wired sensor into the barrier, place this into the patient's oral cavity, remove the barrier with the sensor from the oral cavity, remove the sensor from the barrier, and end with disinfecting the sensor. At this time, sensors cannot withstand heat sterilization or immersion in a high-level disinfectant. Therefore, at a minimum, it is recommended to use a plastic barrier for each sensor, covering the sensor and the top part of the attached cable.

13. C: The dental team should avoid asking any patient questions about disabilities that are unrelated to the care the patient is receiving at the dental clinic to prevent stigmatization of the patient and his or her disability. When working with visually impaired patients, the dental assistant should always inform the patient when they are entering and exiting the treatment as well as steps in the procedure. For hearing-impaired patients, the patient can choose how to communicate with the dental team—options include interpreters, sign language, assistive technology, or written instructions.

14. B: The correct method for disinfecting phosphor storage plates (PSPs) is for the dental radiographer to remove the PSP from the patient's oral cavity with gloved hands. Next, the dental radiographer removes the barrier without touching the PSP to prevent cross contamination and then disinfects the PSP. The PSP is now ready to be placed into the PSP scanner.

15. C: The selector button is located inside the control panel. The selector button is used to select the factors that regulate the x-ray beam. The milliamperage (mA) is how much electrical current goes through the tungsten filament and the mA selector regulates the number of electrons that are produced. The kilovoltage (kVp) selector controls the degree of penetration of the x-ray beam. The exposure button controls the exposure time and is measured in impulses, which are fractions of a second. The master switch is also located within the control panel and turns the machine on and off. The x-ray machine does not produce radiation in the "on" position unless the exposure button is being used. A light located on the control panel indicates if radiation is being produced. Orange indicates the machine is safe and red indicates that radiation is being produced.

16. A: The mounting and labeling of digital images are similar to those of conventional images. The dental auxiliary will be able to move the images around on the computer screen to allow for placement into the correct areas if needed. If digital images are requested by a second dental office, they can be sent electronically so there is no need to print out the images or place them in any type of physical mount. Each set of digital images will be linked to a specific patient, so their full name, birthdate, and address will be noted. The dental axillary who exposed the images should be noted as well as the doctor who requested the images.

17. A: When considering which type of collimator is best in the field of dentistry, the rectangular collimator is the answer. This is because this collimator is the best at reducing excess radiation to the patient because it is shaped the same as the image receptor, so there is less excess radiation that strikes the image receptor. When a circular collimator is used, there is more excess radiation that strikes the patient's skin, and the cone-shaped collimator is no longer used in dentistry due to the excess secondary or scatter radiation that is produced when the radiation strikes the plastic on the cone.

18. C: The hamulus is a small, hook-like projection of bone that is found distal to the maxillary tuberosity. Because of its location, the structure will be shown in maxillary molar periapical images only. The lingual foramen is found in mandibular incisor periapical images, the median palatine suture is located in the maxillary central periapical image, and the mental ridge may be viewed in mandibular central and canine periapical images.

19. D: In dentistry, impulses are used to measure the length of time a patient is exposed to radiation. An impulse is equal to 1/100 of a second, so it is important to know that these two terms, impulse and second, are not interchangeable because an impulse is much shorter than a second.

20. C: Secondary radiation, commonly referred to as scatter radiation, is a type of radiation that is created when primary radiation or the radiation that comes out of the tubehead interacts with matter. This could happen when the primary beam strikes the patient and then deflects towards the dental auxiliary taking the radiographs. There is certain protocol the dental auxiliary must follow to prevent exposure to excess secondary or scatter radiation.

21. D: In dental imaging, the dental radiographer will find that a fair number of disposable items are acceptable for use. Disposable items prevent the chances of cross contamination. These items, also referred to as single-use devices, must be disposed of after a single use. This may result in more waste for the dental office, but this is a valuable trade-off for patient safety.

22. D: There are three stages of dental imaging (before, during, and after), each with their own infection control practices. Before the patient is seen, the dental radiographer should prepare the treatment area, equipment, and supplies and then seat the patient. This includes opening the items and equipment needed for that patient's treatment. Following patient exposure is when the dental radiographer would remove any barriers from the PSPs or wired sensors and disinfect those items to prepare them for the next patient as well as wipe down the patient apron.

23. A: The lingual foramen is an example of an anatomical structure found within the skull that will be present on a mandibular dental image. This structure is a hole in the bone that allows for nerves to pass through, therefore allowing x-rays to pass through and strike the image receptor turning the area black. The incisive foramen and median palatine structures are structures that are present on the maxillary arch and will show on maxillary periapicals. The coronoid process is a mandibular structure that is part of the mandible. Due to its placement, it is shown on the maxillary molar image.

24. C: When viewing dental radiographs, the anatomical landmark that can assist you in mounting the maxillary central periapical is the median palatine suture. The mental ridge is commonly associated with the mandibular periapical. The coronoid process is also associated with the maxilla; however, it is seen usually in the posterior of the mouth rather than in the anterior region of the mouth. The external oblique is associated with the mandible and is oftentimes seen in a molar bitewing radiograph.

25. A: When finished with all radiographic exposures, the patient apron cannot be removed aseptically from the patient by removing it with contaminated gloves. When wearing contaminated gloves, touching any surface will also contaminate this surface. Contaminated gloves should be removed and discarded following the exposure of the final dental image. Immediately following, the hands should be washed and dried. At this time, the patient apron can be removed from the patient and properly disinfected at a convenient time for the dental staff member.

26. B: Storage phosphor imaging is a type of indirect imaging, where the image receptor is not physically connected to a computer or monitoring device. In this type of imaging, a phosphor-coated plate is used to record images; the plates are then placed inside of a computer that records the image and then erases them from the plates, allowing them to be used again and again.

27. C: The 16-inch position-indicating device (PID) is more effective in reducing patient exposure than the other sizes listed. This stems from the fact that the use of the long-cone technique, which requires the use of a 16-inch PID, increases the source-to-receptor distance and reduces skin exposure to dental radiography patients.

28. C: The only statement that is true is the following: "If a lead barrier is not available for the dental radiographer to stand behind, they should stand at a right angle to the beam." The dental radiographer should never stand within six feet of the position-indicating device (PID) during exposure, nor should he or she ever be in the area of the direct beam.

29. D: The bisecting angle technique can be used with any length position-indicating device (PID). Although the bisecting angle technique is often called the "short-cone technique," the long PID can also be used with this technique, as long as the primary beam is directed toward the imaginary bisector dividing the long axis of the tooth and the image receptor.

30. D: The median palatine suture is part of the anatomy in the upper arch that is visible on a maxillary periapical image. This is a location where the two bones that form the roof of the mouth come together, leaving a very thin line that will appear black on a dental image in an area that is otherwise white. The mental foramen is a hole that is found on the lower arch that allows for nerves to pass through and supply the teeth with sensation. The genial tubercles are small bumps of bone that allow for muscles to attach to the lower arch, and the mastoid process is part of the mandible and will be visible in a mandibular periapical image.

31. C: The dental imaging team must have an exposure management plan that identifies the types of procedures that could lead to potential exposures. The dental practice must then make available the PPE that the dental team must wear when participating in those procedures. This will minimize exposure and prevent cross contamination.

32. C: In reference to the properties of the dental x-ray wavelength, the following statement is TRUE: The shorter the wavelength of the x-ray, the greater is its energy. The other statements are false.

33. B: Distortion and overlapping of normal anatomy are caused by the patient's jaws being positioned outside of the focal trough. Although manufacturers of panoramic units are responsible for setting the perimeters of the average-size (focal trough) jaw, most patients' jaw size falls into this average category. Proper positioning of the patient prior to exposure is essential in reducing distortion and overlapping. The intention is to have the patient's jaw positioned within the focal trough of the panoramic unit.

34. A: There are 3 primary components to an x-ray machine: the tubehead, the extension arm, and the control panel. The tubehead is the location of the x-ray tube. The x-ray tube is the place where the x-rays are produced. The x-ray tube is about 6 inches long and allows for electrons to flow through the cathode and the anode. The tubehead is metal and filled with oil that helps to insulate the x-ray tube to prevent it from overheating. The oil also acts to absorb most of the radiation that is produced, allowing only 1% to leave the machine and be directed at the patient. The tubehead is sealed with leaded glass or an aluminum product that prevents radiation from leaking out.

35. A: A full mouth survey (FMX) is used in conjunction with a clinical dental examination. It is a type of intraoral radiograph procedure. A FMX includes 14 periapical views and generally 4 bitewings. New patients should have a full mouth series and this should be repeated as needed depending upon the need to follow up on ongoing conditions or to check for new issues. If the dentist needs to see different views of the structures found within a standard FMX, they will ask the dental team to capture those images. The dental team must always wait for the dentist to make those final decisions.

36. C: The x-rays produced in dentistry have short wavelengths and high frequency (and thus, high energy). When the x-rays contact the outer surface of the patient's skin, they will pass through those tissues and the tissues of the skull to strike the image receptor and capture the structures the dental team needs to see to make an accurate diagnosis. These x-rays are ionizing (i.e., they can cause an electron to be dislodged from a previously stable atom) and can cause damage to the cellular structures of the body, so it is imperative that the dental team take appropriate safety precautions for the patient and themselves.

37. C: When the dentist needs to obtain a detailed view of the ramus area, and, more specifically, a potential fracture of the condylar neck of the mandible, a reverse town projection will be requested. In this projection, the cassette is placed vertically, with the patient facing the cassette, forehead touching the cassette with the chin tilted away, and the mouth open as wide as the patient allows for. The central ray is directed perpendicular to the cassette, originating at the back of the cranium.

38. A: During pregnancy, the adverse health effects of radiation exposure to the fetus are dependent upon the amount of radiation and the timing of the exposure. Fetuses are most sensitive to radiation during weeks 2-15. This is the time when the fetus is made up of cells only. Damage during this period may interfere with normal development of organs; however, because the mother absorbs most of the radiation, it is less likely that birth defects will occur from occupational exposure. A larger risk will occur if the mother inhales radioactive material or receives a very high dose of radiation. A higher dose of radiation would be the equivalent of 500 chest x-rays. Birth defects are even less likely to occur after the 26th week of pregnancy because the baby is fully formed.

39. A: The lingual foramen is a feature of the jaw and, due to its location on the human skull, it will be present on the mandibular central periapical. Because of its structure, it will appear as a black or radiolucent area unless it is filled in by bone. This is an area that allows for soft tissue to move through the bone. The mental foramen is a structure that is found on the mandibular premolar image, the mandibular foramen is found on the mandibular molar image, and the incisive foramen is found on the maxillary central image.

40. C: During intraoral radiography exposure, if the central ray of the beam is not centered on the image receptor, a cone cut will be seen in the resulting image. If part of the image receptor is not penetrated by the primary beam, this portion of the receptor will be unaffected by the exposure. Overlapping will occur if the central x-ray is not aimed between the teeth; elongation will occur if there is not enough vertical angulation used; and ghost imaging is an error that occurs during panoramic imaging if the dental team neglects to have the patient remove earrings, glasses, and piercings found in the head and neck region.

41. A: If a dental image has fewer shades of gray, the image produced has high contrast. If an image has low contrast evident within the processed radiograph, there will be many shades of gray instead of just black and white. Many dental providers prefer a radiograph with low contrast because it enables them to differentiate between periapical and periodontal disease.

42. A: When a low kilovolt peak setting is used, the resulting image will have the greatest contrast. This is because with a low kilovolt setting, the x-rays are not moving as fast. When they strike the image receptor, they are not able to penetrate as many structures and the image has a higher contrast. If the kilovolt setting were increased, the x-rays would move faster and the resulting image would have a lower contrast due to the ability of the x-rays to penetrate more objects.

43. C: The kilovolt peak selector is used to control the penetrating power of the x-ray beam. The tube head encompasses the dental tube that contains the anode, cathode, filament circuit, and tungsten target, which are all part of the process of the creation of the energy needed to produce x-rays. The tungsten filament is the area of the cathode where the thermionic emission of the energy created gathers together.

44. D: When foreshortening is present on a dental image, the dental auxiliary needs to decrease the amount of vertical angulation used in order to correct this. When this is done, the structures on the image will appear in their realistic dimensions. If vertical angulations are further increased, this will result in the image becoming more foreshortened and less diagnostic.

45. A: The electrons that are produced at the tungsten filament on the cathode side of the dental tubehead turn into actual x-rays when they strike the tungsten target, which is located on the anode or the positive side of the tubehead.

46. C: Incipient occlusal describes the type of decay that is just starting in the surface of a tooth and has not worked through the deeper layers of the tooth structure. This type of decay can be caused by eating snacks with high amounts of carbohydrates, by drinking carbonated and/or sugary beverages, and by limited or no flossing. If this type of decay is diagnosed early, the dental team can work with the patient to reduce it. If it is not diagnosed, it will progress to further stages of decay.

47. C: External resorption is a process in which the tissues of the tooth are destroyed. It is referred to as external because this happens from the outside of the tooth. This can be caused by a number of factors, which can then become part of diagnosing the condition. It is visible in dental radiographs: The tooth will appear different and will have dark, radiolucent areas that should be light or radiopaque.

48. B: The standard size image receptor that is used on adults is size 2, but when an adult is present for anterior radiographs, and when that adult has a narrow arch, the dental auxiliary may select a size 1 image receptor for the anterior periapical images. This will allow the dental auxiliary to better place the image receptor behind the required structures and a higher quality image will be captured.

49. C: A dental assistant is considered a category 1 for occupational exposure risk. Any blood or bodily fluids, including saliva, are considered dangerous or infectious. It is impossible to determine who is carrying any sort of infectious disease and each person is considered capable of transmitting certain diseases, such as human immunodeficiency virus (HIV) and hepatitis B virus (HBV). Standard precautions should be followed at all times to protect the health care worker as well as the patient. If an exposure occurs, it is reasonable to ask the patient to submit to blood testing but it cannot be done without the patient's consent. The employee should be advised to obtain blood testing but it cannot be mandated. Proper documentation of the incident is mandatory according to OSHA's bloodborne pathogens (BBP) standard. A written plan must be in place for dealing with occupational exposures. Documentation must include the route of exposure, how the incident occurred, and the source individual and the employee involved.

50. B: A periapical radiograph is an example of an intraoral image. This is used to show the entire tooth structure from the crown to the occlusal surface. It extends about 2-3 mm from the apex to include the periapical bone (jaw). Periapical images are used in the diagnosis of issues with tooth formation and conditions relating to the tooth, root, or bone. Periapical images are used frequently for endodontic treatment as well as oral surgery. The dental assistant must master the technique of paralleling. This is a technique used to obtain high-quality images that are not distorted. The receptor is positioned parallel to the long axis of the tooth and the patient's maxillary occlusal plane must be parallel to the floor. The x-ray beam is then positioned perpendicular to the long axis of the tooth.

51. B: Density can be defined as the overall darkness or blackness of an image receptor. When an image receptor is very dark or black, it is said to have a high density. When an image receptor is lighter, it is said to have a low density. A density that is not too dark or too light is desirable in dentistry in order to show the most structures on the resulting dental radiograph.

52. A: When the image receptor and the image being radiographed, commonly the tooth in dentistry, are placed close together, enlargement of the oral structures is minimized. It is not always possible to place the image receptor and the tooth close together due to the anatomy of the mouth, but when it is possible, this is the desirable method to use.

53. B: Disinfection is the cleaning process that kills or removes some or most of the microbes on a given item or surface, but not all of them (for instance, spores are not killed in the disinfection process and require sterilization). Disinfection is used in the dental operatory room after each patient. Sterilization is then required for semicritical items that enter the patient's mouth and contact the oral mucosa.

54. B: It is acceptable to request that a patient transfer to a different practice if the patient will not allow the dental team to take dental images. Dental images are something that the dentist needs in order to see the full structure of the teeth and any conditions that would otherwise not be visible without these images. It is recommended that a dental office maintain patient records indefinitely. Many offices choose to scan records into their electronic software and then properly dispose of the physical records to reduce the storage space required for patient records. Patients have the right to request their medical, dental, and financial records at any time. They can work with their dental office to complete a records release form to allow for the transfer. This is a requirement regardless of the patient's financial status or if he or she owes the practice money. When it comes to dental images, these should be taken only when a patient's oral status indicates a need. Dental teams should avoid capturing dental images on a standard cycle or based on when insurance will cover the imaging cost. This helps prevent unnecessary radiation exposure to patients.

55. A: Using a PSP is an example of indirect digital imaging. The dental radiographer will place the PSP in the patient's mouth, expose it with radiation, remove the PSP, and then place it in a processing machine, which will then transfer the image to a computer monitor.

56. A: There are several protocols in place for the dental radiographer to follow to prevent disease transmission. These include removing all PPE before leaving a treatment room following any treatments, including the collection of dental images. The dental radiographer must always ensure that hand hygiene is completed before donning gloves and after glove removal. The dental radiographer and the entire dental team should follow standard precautions for uninfected patients, and they should follow heightened precautions for patients with known infectious diseases. There is no need for a patient to remain seated in the dental operatory following completion of any treatment.

57. D: An extension cone paralleling device is considered a semicritical instrument. Like all other dental instruments, it must be precleaned before starting the disinfection and sterilization process. If they are heat stable, semicritical instruments must be sterilized by heat because it is the most effective sterilization method. Using an immersion disinfectant or sterilant including ortho-phthalaldehyde for the disinfectant contact time is not an acceptable method and will not provide a sterile result.

58. B: When viewing an intruded tooth on a dental image, the tooth is seen further up into the tooth socket compared to normal teeth. This condition occurs when there is trauma or force that pushes the tooth up into the bone. The tooth can remain alive, or it may have to be extracted, which will be diagnosed by the dentist upon viewing the image.

59. A: Handwashing is one of the best ways to control infection. Hands should be thoroughly washed before and after putting on gloves. The first handwash of the day should involve the use of a nail brush in order to make sure all bacteria and other microbials have been removed. Any time hands are visibly soiled, soap and water should be used prior to using an alcohol-based hand sanitizer. Alcohol-based hand gel, foam, or rinses are acceptable to use at other times and are quite effective in removing or reducing microbial flora. A concentration of 60-95% is effective. Higher concentrations are not more effective and in fact may be damaging to the skin. It is important to follow instructions for use in order for the hand gel to be most effective. Proper handwashing involves removal of all jewelry, lathering with soap and water for at least 10 seconds, and rinsing with cool water to help close the pores on the hands.

60. D: A dental image with high contrast will have areas of black and with few shades of gray. This is due to the slow-moving x-rays not being able to pass through as many facial and dental structures that produce this type of image. The milliamperage dial is the setting that would affect the overall darkness or lightness of an image receptor.

61. A: When a circular position indicator device (PID) is used, the circular collimator found within the tubehead will restrict the size of the x-ray beam to 2.75 inches in diameter when it strikes the patients face. This is important because it allows for only parts of the patient's face to be exposed and prevents any unnecessary radiation exposure to other areas of the patient.

62. A: The *maximum accumulated lifetime dose* for healthcare workers is calculated as (*N*-18) x 5 rem/year. *N* refers to the worker's age in years, and rem (roentgen equivalent in man) is the unit of measurement set forth by the National Council on Radiation Protection and Measurement for those individuals that are occupationally exposed to radiation. The 5 rem level indicates that level in which no long-term effects were seen per year.

63. A: All dental radiographs are the legal property of the dentist. Patients do have the right to obtain copies of their radiographs for purposes such as transferring to a new dentist or seeing a specialist such as an orthodontist. Original radiographs should never be given to a patient. All dental records should be kept indefinitely for legal purposes. Only copies should be given. The patient can physically take copies of radiographs to the new dentist or they can be mailed once contact information is provided. Digital radiographs can be e-mailed electronically to a new dentist or to a specialist. Legal requirements for patient confidentiality must be adhered to. Digital images may require encryption if the public Internet is used. The patient should also sign a release in regard to the transfer of dental radiographs, and a notation should be made in the patient's record regarding this issue.

64. C: Exposure to radiation can be acute or chronic. Acute exposure would happen when a large dose of radiation is given at one time. An example of this would be an accident at a nuclear plant. Chronic exposure is small amounts of radiation delivered over a longer period of time. Some organs are more at risk for damage than others. The lens of the eye used to be considered a critical organ at risk for damage due to chronic exposure but experts no longer believe this. However, chronic exposure of radiation to the lens of the eye may result in cataracts. Other critical organs that may be affected by chronic exposure to radiation include bone marrow, which can lead to the development of leukemia, the salivary gland, thyroid gland, and skin, which are all at risk for the development of cancer.

65. C. Stainless steel crowns are often used for children as a way to provide treatment to teeth that will eventually be shed. It is used when so much of the tooth is missing that the dentist cannot restore the tooth with amalgam or composite fillings. It is made of less expensive materials (more translucent) compared to other crowns, allowing for the dental radiographer to have the ability to see through the crown on dental images more so than other crowns and dental materials used in dentistry.

66. C: The lead apron is patient equipment that is classified into the noncritical category of dental instruments. It is a noncritical item because it does not enter the oral cavity, nor does it come into contact with the inside of the mouth or the deep, sterile areas of the body. This item is therefore less susceptible to spreading disease and infection, categorizing it as a noncritical item. This categorization determines how the item must be disinfected.

67. C: When considering infection prevention in dental imaging, standard precautions are used just as they are in all other areas of dentistry. The same infection prevention procedures must be used for all patients. There are no additional infection control precautions or exceptions that should be made for any patient, regardless of his or her medical history. Bloodborne infectious diseases require only standard precautions. Individuals with infectious diseases that are airborne in transmission, such as COVID-19 or active tuberculosis, are not recommended for treatment in dentistry per CDC guidelines; therefore, the added PPE would not be indicated because these patients should not be present in the standard dental setting.

68. D: Incorrect horizontal angulation of the PID results in an overlap seen on a bitewing x-ray. Incorrect vertical angulation, when exposing a bitewing, will result in either the maxillary or mandibular crowns of the teeth being included on the radiograph, but not in an equal ratio. An example of this is evident when the vertical angulation is positioned too high: More of the mandibular crowns and tooth structure will be seen, but there will be a deficit in the complete visibility of the maxillary crowns and surrounding bone. This action creates a bitewing x-ray that may be of no diagnostic value. The opposite will be true if the vertical angulation is positioned too low.

69. A: OSHA and the ADA can provide information regarding what the acceptable or permissible dose a healthcare provider can receive to dental professionals, but it is the National Council on Radiation Protection and Measurement that determines, in fact, the maximum permissible dose allowed for a healthcare provider.

70. B: When the Frankfort plane is too high during the positioning of a patient for a panoramic image, a reversed "smile line" will result. This reversed smile line will curve downward. When positioned correctly, the Frankfort plane will be displayed as a smile line slightly curved upward, indicating the correct direction of the curve of Spee.

71. D: When a patient is present for dental images and they have lingual tori in their mouth, the dental auxiliary needs to be careful not to place the image receptor on top of the tori because this will result in discomfort for the patient. The dental auxiliary needs to place the image receptor on the far side of the tori and then expose the image.

72. B: The use of an aluminum filter in the tubehead prevents low-energy, weak x-rays from exiting the tubehead and striking the patient. If these x-rays were allowed to strike the patient, they have a higher chance of being absorbed by the patient's tissue and potentially causing biological damage to the patient. In dentistry, high-energy, fast-moving x-rays are desirable due to their ability to penetrate oral structures and strike the image receptor in the patient's mouth.

73. C: All of the following would appear radiopaque on a processed dental periapical image EXCEPT a sinus cavity. The tuberosity, the dense alveolar bone, and a metal restoration would appear radiopaque because the x-ray beam would not be able to penetrate, or go through, these substances. Varying degrees of radiopacity would be seen in each of the anatomical areas and metal restorations.

74. A: During x-ray production, the purpose of the step-down transformer is to decrease the voltage from 110 or 220 volts to 3 to 5 volts. This decrease in voltage is necessary in the production of energy that can be used for the production of charged electrons worthy of being discharged through the PID and onto the dental receptor.

75. B: Intermediate-level disinfectants have the correct ingredients in the correct concentrations to kill microbes, including tuberculosis, from dental surfaces. These are used in areas such as the patient chair, light handles, and position indicator devices; they must be used in the correct amounts in these areas in order to be effective.

76. D: The Frankfurt plane can be defined as the plane formed by the opening of the ear canal and the bottom of the eye socket. This is commonly used in dentistry as an indicator for proper head positioning and can be a helpful tool to use when exposing both extraoral and intraoral images.

77. C: This statement, "Primary radiation is created when the secondary radiation interacts with matter," is false because it is primary radiation that is emitted from the target of the x-ray tube. The other statements are true.

78. B: If the dental radiographer receives an injury that goes through all skin layers or receives a splash of fluid to the eyes, he or she should stop the procedure immediately. The next steps would be to wash the puncture area with soap and water or flush the eyes with water. Then, the injured individual should report the injury to the appropriate person in their dental office for documentation and next steps. In the case of needle punctures post–patient use, blood testing may be requested of the patient to confirm that there are no bloodborne infections that the dental radiographer may have been exposed to.

79. C: Overlapping is an exposure error that occurs on image receptors when the dental auxiliary does not aim the central ray perpendicular to the teeth being exposed. When this is aimed incorrectly, the central ray causes the teeth to appear overlapped or on top of one another, making it impossible to see if there are any conditions occurring interproximally.

80. A: A periapical abscess is an area of infection caused by the destruction of the pulp tissue. Once the pulp tissue dies, it needs to be removed through a root canal procedure or it will spill out from the tooth through the foramen. When this happens, the dead tissue that leaves through the foramen will destroy the surrounding bone, leading to the development of destroyed soft tissue, which is viewable on a dental radiograph.

RHS Practice Test #2

1. During panoramic positioning of the patient, if the patient's chin is positioned too low, the following will be seen on the processed radiograph:

a. a smile line curved downward.
b. open contact on the posterior teeth.
c. detail in the anterior apical regions.
d. the absence of the patient's condyles in the correct anatomical position.

2. All of the following are accurate statements regarding hand hygiene under dental gloves EXCEPT:

a. The dental radiographer's fingernails should be short enough so that they do not interfere with the placement and removal of dental gloves.
b. Chipped nail polish found on the fingernails of the dental radiographer may increase the number of bacteria found in those areas.
c. Rings should be avoided because the skin underneath them contains more bacteria and viruses compared to skin in other areas without rings.
d. Petroleum-based lotions are found to be the most beneficial for dental radiographers to use under gloves, allowing for the lotion to have the proper contact time with the skin.

3. Which one of the following is accurate about direct digital imaging?

a. A sensor is placed in the mouth, it is exposed to radiation, and an image immediately appears on a monitor for viewing.
b. A sensor is placed in the mouth, it is exposed to radiation, it is processed by a scanner, and the image is emailed to the user for viewing.
c. A sensor is used to record the image, the image is sent to a central processor for processing, and then it will be viewable by the dental team.
d. A sensor is placed in the mouth, it is exposed to radiation and placed in the processing machine, the image is edited, and then the image will appear ready for viewing.

4. All of the following statements regarding the somatic effect of radiation are TRUE, EXCEPT:

a. Damage caused by radiation from somatic effects is passed on to future generations.
b. X-rays can damage somatic tissues.
c. One possible somatic effect of radiation is cancer.
d. X-rays affect somatic cells.

5. Which of the following is an accurate description of ionization?

a. The pairing of electrons and protons to create ions.
b. The creation of stable atoms due to radiation striking the nucleus of an ion.
c. The process of particulate radiation striking a cell and destroying the DNA of that cell.
d. The process of converting stable atoms into ions.

6. Tomography can be best described as:

a. the production of a clear, crisp image.
b. the process of imaging a desired structure while blurring of other areas.
c. capturing the upper arch of the oral cavity and projecting it over the lower arch.
d. the process of capturing the coronal portion of each erupted tooth.

7. Which one of the following is an example of an acceptable disinfection technique used in dental imaging?

a. Leaving patient care items in their packaging until they are ready for use
b. Using low-level disinfectants to disinfect clinical contact surfaces
c. Using an immersion sterilant for a heat-stable beam alignment device
d. Disinfecting the radiographic patient apron for patient use at the end of the day

8. When preparing the dental imaging area for patient care, which one of the following is an accurate statement?

a. The dental assistant should retrieve all items including beam alignment devices, open all packages, and lay out the items in the imaging area to allow for decreased imaging time.
b. The radiographic imager should place barriers over radiographic equipment including the exposure button and control panel because there are often hard-to-reach areas that may create reservoirs for pathogens and other microbes.
c. Barriers are not recommended for use in areas where dental images are captured due to the heat generation from the dental radiographic machines that may cause any barriers being used to have the potential to melt to the equipment or become compromised.
d. Due to the nature of dental imaging and the limited amounts of mucosa contact, spray, and spatter, PPE is not required for the dental radiographer; therefore, it does not need to be stocked in the dental imaging area.

9. Which statement best describes the effects of long-term low-dose radiation exposure?

a. The effect of long-term low-dose radiation exposure will cause genetic defects for both men and women in their childbearing years
b. The effect of long-term low-dose radiation exposure will cause cancer
c. The effect of long-term low-dose radiation exposure can cause changes at the cellular level in the human body that would be observed within 2 years
d. The effect of long-term low-dose radiation exposure can cause changes at the cellular level in the human body that would not be observed for many years

10. The difference between acute radiation exposure and chronic radiation exposure is:

a. the type of radiation received.
b. the type of scattered radiation received.
c. the amount of radiation received and the time frame in which it is absorbed.
d. the type of wavelengths creating the exposure

11. Identify the density and contrast of a dental image produced using a high kilovolt or kV setting:

a. High density; low contrast.
b. High density; high contrast.
c. Low density; low contrast.
d. Low density; high contrast.

12. To prevent cross contamination from a used sensor holder, which one of the following must be avoided?

a. Place the used/contaminated sensor holder into a secure container for transport to the instrument processing area.
b. Have separate locations for receiving/cleaning, prepping/packaging, and sterilizing/storing instruments in the instrument processing area.
c. Forgo precleaning practices on the sensor holder including hand scrubbing, automated washing, or the use of an ultrasonic machine if the dental radiographer does not see any debris on the item.
d. If manual cleaning is not able to be performed immediately following use, the dental radiographer can soak the item in an acceptable solution to prevent the drying of debris onto the item.

13. Which one of the following will appear on dental images as white restorations that commonly appear in the posterior area of the mouth and are examples of indirect restorations?

a. Amalgam restorations
b. Gold crowns
c. Composite restorations
d. Porcelain crowns

14. When describing the long axis of a tooth when referring to the paralleling technique, which of the following statements is TRUE?

a. The long axis can be seen on each tooth.
b. The long axis of the tooth divides it into equal thirds.
c. The long axis of the tooth divides it into equal halves.
d. The long axis of the tooth divides it into equal sections; one section contains only the crown of the tooth, and the other section contains only the root of the tooth.

15. When viewing dental images, which anatomical landmark can assist you in identifying the molar bitewing?

a. The maxillary sinus.
b. The mandibular canal.
c. The mental foramen.
d. The external oblique.

16. A reversed smile line observed on a panoramic image is likely due to:

a. Position of the patient's chin is too high
b. Position of the patient's chin is too low
c. The patient's spine is not straight
d. The patient's lips were not closed during imaging

17. Which of the following is the device that restricts the size and shape of the x-ray beam?

a. Aluminum filter
b. Lead collimator
c. Tungsten target
d. Molybdenum focusing cup.

18. If the kilovolt peak (kVp) setting is lowered, how will this affect the resulting image?

a. The image will have a higher contrast
b. The image will show areas of black and white with many shades of gray between them
c. The image will have elongation and stretched roots
d. The image will be non-diagnosable due to extreme darkness or blackness

19. If a dental x-ray tube head has a faulty seal, the following will result:

a. the x-ray unit will not emit radiation/energy to successfully capture a dental image.
b. leakage of radiation.
c. the electrical system of the dental radiography unit will sound an alarm.
d. the x-ray unit will not turn on.

20. What is the most likely reason for a dental radiographer to receive a reading on their personal radiation monitoring device?

a. Failure of the dental radiographer in following the rules of working with radiation, to include not wearing the badge outside of the clinic/practice.
b. Non-functioning digital sensor.
c. Uncooperative patients.
d. Faulty radiation-monitoring device.

21. Which of the following is a main disadvantage of using digital imaging in dentistry?

a. The gray-scale resolution.
b. The speed of viewing images.
c. The amount of radiation that a patient is exposed to.
d. The sensor size and thickness.

22. Which of the following is a true statement regarding the use of patient aprons and thyroid collars?

a. The use of patient aprons and thyroid collars will prevent cancer from developing in the thyroid gland.
b. The apron should cover from the neck to just above the patient's knees.
c. Patient aprons should be cleaned thoroughly and folded in thirds between patient use.
d. The thyroid collar is optional for older adults past childbearing years.

23. Which one of the following is the correct procedure when using phosphor storage plates (PSPs)?

a. Gather the PSPs, place each PSP in a barrier, capture the images, remove each PSP from its barrier, and allow each PSP to drop into a cup that will be used for transporting the plates to the scanner once all images have been obtained.
b. Collect the PSPs required for the patient, disinfect each PSP, place the PSPs into the patient's oral cavity to capture the image with no barrier, remove the PSPs, disinfect them again, and transport them to the scanner for processing.
c. Place each PSP in a scanner for disinfection prior to use, collect the PSPs needed for patient care, place each PSP in a barrier, capture the image, remove the barrier, place the PSPs in the scanner to capture the image, and then store the PSPs for future use.
d. Collect the PSPs while setting up the treatment room, disinfect each PSP, allow each one to dry, place the PSPs in a barrier, use the PSPs to capture the images, remove the barriers with the PSPs from the oral cavity, remove the PSPs from the barriers, place each PSP into a scanning disinfectant solution, and place into the PSP scanner.

24. Which of the following will appear the most radiopaque on a dental radiograph?

a. Composite restorations.
b. Amalgam restorations.
c. Gutta percha.
d. Porcelain crowns.

25. When is it acceptable to sterilize an extension cone paralleling (XCP) device without the use of packaging?

a. When an XCP device is processed through the chemiclave, which will allow for a chemical residue to remain on the item that prevents contamination until the item can be used, allowing for short term, unpackaged storage.
b. When a dental office is out of the packaging material that is needed to properly package and sterilize the XCP device. It can be stored for a period of up to 7 days before it must be packaged and resterilized.
c. An XCP device must be packaged before sterilization to maintain its sterility afterward.
d. When the XCP device will be transferred to the point of use immediately following sterilization and can be done so in an aseptic manner.

26. Which one of the following is a radiation hazard that emerges from the soil as a colorless and odorless gas that can cause lung cancer?

a. Fallout radiation
b. Cosmic energy
c. Radon
d. UV radiation

27. Which of the following choices is TRUE regarding chronic radiation exposure?

a. This type of radiation exposure is a risk to dental staff that process dental radiographs.
b. Chronic radiation exposure will not be passed on to future generations.
c. This type of exposure can be easily linked to the source.
d. Exposure to radiation from a nuclear power plant leak is an example of chronic radiation exposure.

28. Which one of the following is correct regarding infection control practices in dental imaging and photostimulable phosphor plates (PSPs)

a. When PSPs are removed from the mouth, they are contaminated and should be removed with gloved hands.
b. It is a common infection control practice for the dental radiographer to ask the patient to remove the PSP from the mouth after the receptor has been exposed to radiation in order to minimize the radiographer's contact with the patient's oral mucosa.
c. Barriers are uncommonly used with PSPs due to the antimicrobial properties of the imaging sensors.
d. PSPs are reusable and do not need barriers because the PSP processing machine disinfects each plate as it pulls the image off the PSP.

29. Which one of the following is accurate regarding housekeeping surfaces found in the dental radiography area of the dental office?

a. Housekeeping surfaces have a high risk of disease transmission.
b. Housekeeping surfaces have to be decontaminated at the same level as clinical contact surfaces.
c. An example of a housekeeping surface is the floor.
d. Housekeeping surfaces must be cleaned after each patient encounter.

30. The maximum permissible dose of occupational radiation exposure for dental staff allowed in a year is:

a. 100 mrem.
b. 3 Roentgens.
c. 5 rem.
d. 6 rad.

31. Which one of the following can be described as the projection of bone that is found behind the upper last-erupted tooth?

a. Nutrient canal
b. Zygomatic process of the maxilla
c. Hamulus
d. Anterior nasal spine

32. What is the minimum proper distance for the operator to stand away from the x-ray beam to minimize exposure?

a. 2 feet
b. 4 feet
c. 6 feet
d. 8 feet

33. The density of a dental image is directly associated with which setting?

a. exposure time.
b. the milliamp (mA) setting.
c. the kilovolt peak (kVp) setting.
d. the impulse setting.

34. What is the federal requirement regarding the thickness of the aluminum filter on an x-ray machine operating at 70 kVp or greater?

a. The thickness of the aluminum filtration must be 2.0 mm.
b. The thickness of the aluminum filtration must be 3.0 mm.
c. The thickness of the aluminum filtration must be 4.0 mm.
d. The thickness of the aluminum filtration must be 2.5 mm.

35. Dental radiographers with which one of the following conditions should avoid direct patient care for a predetermined period to reduce the chance of disease transmission?

a. Bacterial sinus infection
b. Herpes simplex type 1 on the lips
c. Open lesions on the hands
d. Cold sores on the roof of the mouth

36. Cone-beam computed tomography (CBCT) allows for which feature that traditional dental panoramic imagery cannot?

a. The ability to see both arches.
b. The ability to distinguish between the types of soft tissues present.
c. The ability to view impacted wisdom teeth.
d. The ability to view the anatomy of the skull.

37. Which one of the following terms can be described as the areas of a dental image that appear white or lighter in color due to x-ray beams becoming lodged in dense structures and not being able to strike the image receptor?

a. Radiopaque
b. High density
c. Radiolucent
d. Low contrast

38. Which one of the following is the correct image to use to look for mesial decay on tooth #29?

a. Molar periapical
b. Molar bitewing
c. Premolar periapical
d. Premolar bitewing

39. Which of the following causes foreshortening?

a. Inadequate vertical angle.
b. Inadequate horizontal angle.
c. Too much vertical angle.
d. Incomplete coverage of the image receptor.

40. Which dental imaging technique can be used to reduce radiation exposure to the eye?

a. bisecting angle technique.
b. beam cone technique.
c. paralleling technique.
d. occlusal technique.

41. A young patient is having difficulty holding still for dental imaging. What is the recommended next step for the dental assistant to take?

a. Try again next appointment
b. Ask the parent to have the child sit on his or her lap with both covered by the patient apron
c. Ask the dentist to hold the child
d. Stand next to the child and hold the sensor in place until the x-rays are completed

42. An operator should become concerned if their weekly dosage of radiation exceeds:

a. 5 mR.
b. 50 mR.
c. 75 mR.
d. 100 mR.

43. Which one of the following is the standard measure for the highest amount of radiation that an individual can be exposed to prior to intervening action being taken?

a. As low as reasonably achievable (ALARA) principle
b. Cumulative occupational dose (COD)
c. Maximum permissible dose (MPD)
d. Radiation Control for Health and Safety Act Maximum (RCHSAM)

44. After using an extension cone paralleling device, it is precleaned, packaged, and sterilized. Which one of the following is the only way to guarantee that sterilization has occurred after the item has completed the sterilization cycle?

a. The use of a biological indicator placed within the instrument load and processed for results
b. The assessment of the physical indicator that is often found on the instrument packaging or sterilization tape
c. The chemical monitoring indicators that can be placed within each sterilization package
d. The report that is generated from each load identifying the time, temperature, and pressure to which items were exposed to for each sterilization cycle

45. Which one of the following is an example of a semicritical item used in dental imaging?

a. Blood pressure cuff
b. Cotton roll used to stabilize a receptor
c. XCP device
d. Position indicator device

46. The patient apron is classified as what type of item when it comes to its cleaning and processing?

a. noncritical
b. semicritical
c. patient critical
d. dentist critical

47. Which one of the following is the correct procedure to follow regarding infection control when performing patient dental images with PSPs?

a. After each PSP is removed from the oral cavity, place it in an immersion disinfectant for a minimum of 5 minutes.
b. Wear gloves when removing PSPs or digital sensors from a patient's mouth.
c. When heat sterilizing PSPs, ensure that they are not overlapped in the sterilization machine, which will result in failure to fully sterilize the plates.
d. When using PSPs, after each image is taken, it is required to remove that image from the barrier immediately after processing and wipe the plate with disinfectant. The dental radiographer must not wait until all images have been captured because that will allow for an increased risk of cross contamination.

48. What modification in technique is recommended when the patient has an edentulous space causing a problem with the bite-wing image receptor placement?

a. Replace the bitewing image with a panoramic image.
b. Place a cotton roll in the area of the missing tooth/teeth to stabilize the image receptor.
c. Have the patient hold the image receptor in position with a hemostat.
d. Take a periapical image with a bite-block instead.

49. A properly exposed bitewing image will show all of the following EXCEPT:

a. the crestal bone.
b. maxillary and mandibular crowns.
c. the interproximal areas of the teeth within the image.
d. a periapical radiolucency.

50. When the occlusal plane on an image appears tipped, the error is:

a. that incorrect horizontal angulations were used.
b. that the image is elongated.
c. that the image moved when the patient was biting down.
d. that incorrect vertical angulations were used.

51. Movement of the patient during panoramic exposure will result in:

a. superimposed imagery.
b. darkening of the dental structures.
c. ghost imagery.
d. blurred imagery.

52. Which of the following cell groups of tissue are LEAST likely to be affected by radiation?

a. Oral mucosa
b. Bone marrow
c. Nerve tissue
d. Connective tissue

53. Which one of the following instructions must be adhered to when the dental team is using alcohol-based hand rubs in dental imaging?

a. The dental team must wash their hands with antimicrobial soap prior to the use of alcohol-based hand rubs.
b. When used, the dental team must rub their hands together until the alcohol-based hand rub has been absorbed into the hands.
c. The dental team must rinse their hands following application of alcohol-based hand rubs to remove residual microbes.
d. The dental team must avoid alcohol-based hand rubs that have alcohol concentrations greater than 40% due to the breakdown of the active ingredient over this threshold.

54. Which of the following statements is correct regarding infection control in dental radiography?

a. Intraoral digital sensors must be covered with plastic barrier envelopes to minimize contamination.
b. Digital sensors may be heat sterilized after use.
c. The dental chair does not need to be wiped down if exposing radiographs was the only procedure to take place in the operatory.
d. There is no need to use plastic barriers on digital sensors as long as they are disinfected with a low-level disinfectant after use.

55. The safest place for the dental auxiliary to stand during an exposure would be:

a. 90–135° to the patient.
b. 90–135° to the tubehead.
c. behind the patient.
d. in front of the patient.

56. Which of the following is NOT a disadvantage to digital radiography?

a. Infection control issues
b. Lost images
c. Cost for purchasing digital imaging equipment
d. Training

57. Which one of the following guidelines is false with regard to capturing dental images?

a. The active part of the sensor should be facing the teeth or the oral structure being radiographed.
b. Anterior films should be placed in a vertical layout when possible.
c. The receptor holder should be positioned toward the middle of the mouth to allow for parallelism.
d. The receptor should be placed perpendicular to the teeth or oral structures to accurately capture the geometry of the structure(s).

58. What part of the x-ray machine functions to remove the most dangerous x-rays from reaching both the patient and the operator?

a. Aluminum filter
b. Collimator
c. PID
d. Milliamperage selector

59. Which of the following is an INCORRECT statement regarding the use of digital technologies in dental radiography?

a. The digital sensors used may be wired or wireless depending on the brand and the needs of a dental clinic.
b. In digital imaging, the sensor receives the image information and converts it into a digital image in the computer processing unit.
c. The essential components of a digital imaging system include a source of radiation, a sensor, and a computer.
d. Digital reduces the amount of radiation a patient is exposed to by 10% compared with the historical use of film-based imaging.

60. Which of the following images should include the retromolar pad area found in the dentition?

a. Maxillary premolar periapical.
b. Molar bitewing.
c. Mandibular molar periapical.
d. Maxillary molar periapical.

61. When considering hand hygiene for the dental radiographer, which one of the following is correct?

a. Transient flora is commonly acquired by the dental radiographer during direct patient care activities and can be easily removed with proper hand hygiene.
b. When preparing for dental imaging, the only acceptable method of hand hygiene for the dental radiographer is washing the hands with water and antimicrobial soap.
c. The dental radiographer is responsible for ensuring that all residential flora is removed from the hands before entering the dental imaging area.
d. If the dental radiographer's glove sustains a small tear during dental imaging, he or she should finish the image they are working on, doff gloves, perform hand hygiene, and then don new gloves.

62. Which type of radiation is created when the primary beam comes in contact with any matter?

a. Primary radiation.
b. Secondary radiation.
c. Quandary radiation.
d. Scattered radiation.

63. How does the use of photostimulable storage phosphor (PSP) plates affect digital radiography?

a. PSP plates are the thickest form of sensor and are the most uncomfortable to the patient
b. PSP plates allow for heat sterilization, making infection control easier to manage
c. PSP plates provide slightly more radiation exposure to the patient than historical film-based imaging
d. PSP plates do not offer immediate access to the digital image

64. Which of the following should be done to correct elongation?

a. Increase horizontal angle.
b. Increase vertical angle.
c. Decrease horizontal angle.
d. Decrease vertical angle.

65. When using the paralleling technique during periapical exposure:

a. the receptor and the long axis of the tooth are perpendicular to each other.
b. the receptor and the long axis of the tooth are at right angles to each other.
c. the receptor and the long axis of the tooth are at a 45-degree angle to each other.
d. the receptor and the long axis of the tooth are parallel to each other.

66. The ALARA concept can best be described by which of the following statements?

a. Patient exposure to dental radiation should be maintained to at least as reasonably achievable.
b. Patient exposure to dental radiation should be maintained to as low as the radiation allows.
c. Patient exposure to dental radiation should be maintained to as low as rays are arranged correctly.
d. Patient exposure to dental radiation should be maintained to as low as reasonably achievable.

67. Which one of the following is the correct process when exposing dental images on a patient who is 5 months pregnant?

a. The dental team must use the patient apron during exposure.
b. The dental team should avoid taking dental images on a pregnant patient.
c. There should be no deviation from the standard protocol for pregnant patients.
d. The pregnant patient should be exposed to images from the panoramic machine only.

68. Which of the following refers to the number of wavelengths that pass a given point in a certain amount of time?

a. Propagation.
b. Velocity.
c. Wavelength.
d. Frequency.

69. Which of the following is the correct size of the image receptor that should be used for adult occlusal radiographs?

a. Size 2.
b. Size 4.
c. Size 3.
d. Size 0.

70. When viewing a full mouth series of dental images, which of the following anatomical structures will be found in the center of the maxillary canine periapical?

a. Inverted Y.
b. Hamulus.
c. Zygomatic process.
d. Mental foramen.

71. Identify which of the following cell groups of tissue are MOST likely to be affected by radiation:

a. reproductive cells.
b. muscle tissue.
c. thyroid gland.
d. liver.

72. Disposal of an extracted tooth is considered to be:

a. General waste
b. Toxic waste
c. Infectious waste
d. Hazardous waste

73. During extraoral panoramic dental radiography, what distortion will result when the tongue is not kept in contact with the maxillary palate during exposure?

a. a dark shadow will obscure the apices of the maxillary teeth.
b. a dark shadow will obscure the apices of the mandibular teeth.
c. a dark shadow will obscure the sinuses of the maxillary teeth.
d. a blurred image will obscure the apices of the mandibular teeth.

74. What is the maximum permissible dose (MPD) of radiation for a dental assistant?

a. 5 rem/year
b. 0.5 rem/year
c. 10 rem/year
d. 50 rem/year

75. The Frankfort plane is described as:

a. a plane that passes through the floor of the orbit and to the external auditory meatus.
b. a plane dividing the face into symmetrical left and right hemispheres.
c. a plane that must remain perpendicular to the floor.
d. a plane that must be parallel to the shoulders of the patient.

76. What correction is needed if distal of the cuspid is not present on a bicuspid image?

a. Place the image receptor vertically in the mouth.
b. Direct central ray at center of the image receptor.
c. Decrease vertical angle used on the image.
d. Place the image receptor more anterior in the mouth.

77. Which of the following is a TRUE statement that will aid the assistant in correctly identifying dental images?

a. The mental foramen will appear in the mandibular molar periapical image.
b. The coronoid process will appear in the maxillary molar periapical image.
c. The genial tubercles will appear in the maxillary central periapical image.
d. The tuberosity will appear in the mandibular molar periapical image.

78. Which of the below choices is INCORRECT regarding a high dose of radiation?

a. It may be produced by dental x-rays.
b. It may occur as a result of nuclear weapon use.
c. It may be used in radiation therapy for cancer treatment.
d. It has a short latent period.

79. When using the paralleling technique during intraoral periapical exposure, the receptor should be placed _______________ and _______________.

a. as close as possible to the teeth, near the lingual surface of the teeth.
b. as close as possible to the teeth, near the occlusal surface of the teeth.
c. as far away as possible from the lingual surface of the teeth, near the middle of the mouth.
d. as far away as possible from the lingual surface of the teeth, near the opposite side of the mouth.

80. What is the purpose of a periapical image?

a. To capture the crowns of the teeth to identify occlusal decay
b. To see the teeth and oral structures in three dimensions
c. To view incipient interproximal decay on the molars
d. To capture the full root and coronal structure of the teeth being imaged

Answer Key and Explanations for Test #2

1. D: During panoramic positioning of the patient, if the patient's chin is positioned too low, the patient's condyles are *not* shown in their correct anatomical position. Often, the borders of the ramus and condyles, bilaterally, are seen as being distorted in width and seemingly higher in the cranial cavity than they should be as related to the correct anatomical position of such landmarks.

2. D: Petroleum-based lotions should be avoided or only used at the end of the workday in the dental workplace. These products have been shown to weaken the structure of some gloves, making it easier for bacteria and other microbes to reach the skin underneath the gloves. There are certain lotions recommended for use in dentistry, and the dental radiographer should contact their dental supply representative to learn more about the correct products to use and the best way to use them.

3. A: Direct imaging is used in dentistry and allows the dental team to place a sensor in the patient's mouth, press the exposure button, and have the image immediately appear on a monitor. This allows for quick viewing and diagnosis in everyday use and in emergency situations.

4. A: The only statement that is false in this series of statements is "Damage caused by radiation from somatic effects is passed on to future generations." This statement is false. Dental x-rays are capable of harming somatic tissues and cells, which may result in cancer, but this harm is not inheritable to future offspring.

5. D: Ionization is the process in which stable atoms are disrupted by radiation and ions are created. Ions are charged particles and include the negative electrons that can be ejected from a stable atom after it is struck by radiation.

6. B: Tomography can be described as the process of imaging a desired structure while blurring other areas on an image. This is how panoramic images are produced as well as other types of extraoral projections.

7. A: It is important to leave any patient care items in their packaging until ready for use, which is when the patient is seated in the chair and can watch the dental radiographer open the packaging onto the sterile tray. If an item is opened before the patient is in the chair, there is no way to ensure that the item is clean and sterile, which may lead to undue concern by the patient and possible points of entry for microbes prior to use. This is a common infection control practice for dentistry and the medical field.

8. B: When preparing for patient care, if available, the dental radiographer should place barriers over the dental radiographic equipment. This equipment may have small areas and crevices where microbes can enter, creating hard-to-disinfect areas. The dental assistant should avoid opening any packages until the patient is in the treatment room and can watch the instruments that will be used being opened. When considering the use of PPE, the dental assistant is required to wear gloves during the placement and removal of digital sensors because these are placed directly into the oral cavity. Eye and respiratory protection is also required to be available for the dental assistant to use in every procedure, including dental imaging.

9. D: About half of radiation exposure in the United States occurs because of medical procedures such as x-rays, CT scans, or other types of procedures. Low doses of radiation do not cause an immediate medical or genetic effect. The effects of long-term low-dose radiation exposure are typically not seen for 5-20 years and may manifest as changes in the cellular level in the human body. The main concerns for radiation exposure are cancer and genetic defects. The chances for either to occur are possible but are less likely to occur from low-dose exposure.

10. C: The difference between acute and chronic radiation exposure is the amount of radiation received and the time frame in which it is absorbed. In acute radiation exposure, a large or very high amount of radiation is exposed over a short period of time. This can lead to serious illness. Chronic radiation exposure is an unspecified amount of exposure over a long period of time. The amount of exposure and the overall length of time that the exposure was given will determine if it will cause a lasting effect.

11. A: When a high kilovolt setting is used, the dental tubehead produces x-rays that are moving faster, and when these x-rays strike the image receptor, they cause the resulting image to have a high density and a low contrast. This is because the x-rays are moving faster and are able to penetrate more objects that are in their path. If this were undesirable, the operator could turn down the kilovolt setting, which would reduce the density and increase the contrast.

12. C: It is important for the dental radiographer to preclean all items and instruments in use when capturing dental images, including sensor holders such as the Snap-A-Ray and extension cone paralleling device. If these items are not properly precleaned, they can be placed into a sterilization unit while carrying physical particles on it that can block the effects of the sterilization machine, leading to the potential for cross contamination.

13. B: Gold crowns are examples of indirect restorations that are commonly used in the posterior area of the mouth in dentistry. Because these indirect restorations are made of high-quality materials, they appear white or radiopaque on dental images and can be distinguished from their amalgam counterparts by looking at the borders of the item on the tooth structure in the image.

14. C: With regard to the paralleling technique, the long axis of the tooth divides the tooth into two equal halves. This long axis cannot be seen and must be imagined clinically by the dental radiographer. Through knowledge of dental anatomy and morphology, it must be understood that the roots of the teeth in the oral cavity are specifically angled in the alveolar bone, creating this long axis of the tooth. The only time the tooth is thought of as being divided horizontally between the crown and root will usually be when discussing the identification of the anatomical crown versus the root of the tooth.

15. D: When viewing dental images, the anatomical landmark that can assist you in identifying the molar bitewing is the external oblique. The mental foramen will not assist you in identifying a molar bitewing because this anatomical landmark is found in the periapical region of the mandibular bicuspids. Bitewing radiographs are not to include the apices of the teeth being radiographed; therefore, the mental foramen should not be seen in the bitewing radiograph. The mandibular canal is seen in the mandibular bicuspid or molar periapical, at the area of the apices of the bicuspids and/or molar. A properly positioned bitewing radiograph will not be placed to include the apices of the mandibular teeth. The maxillary sinus will not be included in the molar bitewing because it is an anterior periapical anatomical landmark usually seen in maxillary anterior periapicals.

16. A: Proper positioning of the patient during panoramic imaging is essential to good quality results. The patient should be standing tall with the spine as straight as possible. The patient needs to bite down on the plastic bite block. The midsagittal plane (the imaginary vertical line that divides the face in half equally) is aligned perpendicular to the floor and the Frankfort plane (imaginary horizontal line under the eye and at the top of the ear canal) is aligned parallel with the floor. The patient's tongue should be on the roof of the mouth and the lips should be closed. A reverse smile line where the smile appears to curve downward is due to the position of the chin being too high. An exaggerated smile line where the smile curves upward is due to the chin being positioned too low.

17. B: The lead collimator is a device found inside of the dental tubehead and is used to control the size and the shape of the x-ray beam as it exits the tubehead. This differs from the aluminum filter, which is used to remove the weak or slow-moving x-rays from the x-ray beam. The tungsten target is responsible for providing a surface where the electrons generated by the tungsten filament can collide with to turn into x-rays. The molybdenum focusing cup is a structure that keeps the electrons together before the exposure button is pressed, allowing for the release of the electrons.

18. A: If a kilovolt peak (kVp) setting is lowered, the contrast of an image will increase. The kVp setting controls the speed or how fast the x-rays move through the tubehead and out the position indicator device to the oral structures and the image receptor. If the x-rays are moving too slow, which can happen as the kVp setting is lowered or decreased, this means they are not moving strong enough to penetrate the oral structures including the teeth which will result in a high contrast image or an image that has black and white areas with few shades of gray. This can result in missing pathological conditions and areas of decay in the mouth.

19. B: If a dental x-ray tube head has a faulty seal, radiation leakage will result. Operation of the dental x-ray unit will not be disabled. Quality assurance practices can help to maintain safe operational equipment. In the event that a dental x-ray tube head is thought to have a faulty seal, the unit should immediately be taken out of service and it should be checked out.

20. A: The most likely reason for a dental radiographer to receive a reading on their personal radiation-monitoring device is his or her failure to follow the rules of working with radiation, to include not wearing the badge outside of the clinic/practice. Wearing the badge outside of the clinic exposes the monitoring device to atmospheric radiation that is common in everyday living.

21. D: Digital imaging has many advantages, but one of the few disadvantages is the size and rigidity of the image receptor that is used during this technique. Due to the components that need to be placed in the image receptor, it is thicker than a standard image receptor that is used in conventional radiography. The image receptor is also very rigid, which can produce patient discomfort during exposures.

22. B: A patient apron and thyroid collar are optional protective equipment items that can be used on patients as an extra safety precaution to protect them from ionizing radiation. The patient apron should be positioned so it covers from the neck to just above the patient's knees, covering the reproductive organs. The thyroid collar can either be attached to the apron or can be a separate piece. It should be correctly positioned to cover the area of the thyroid. Patient aprons should never be folded or hung on anything with a sharp edge because this may cause the apron to crack over time. It should be hung on a special hanger or draped over a rod.

23. A: When capturing images with phosphor storage plates (PSPs), it is important to use correct infection control techniques. The correct process is to gather the PSPs, place each PSP into a barrier, capture the images, remove each PSP from its barrier, and allow each PSP to drop into a cup that will be used for transporting the plates to the scanner once all images have been obtained. Barriers are required for use with PSPs because they cannot withstand heat or immersion sterilization. PSPs do not need to be disinfected prior to use because they should already be disinfected, stored, and ready for placement into barriers when needed.

24. B: Amalgam restorations will appear the most radiopaque due to what they are made from. Any material that is made from metal or metal-based elements will appear completely radiopaque because the x-rays are not able to penetrate these items. When viewing composites, porcelain crowns, and gutta percha, these will still appear radiopaque, but not as radiopaque as metallic structures because they do not contain metallic elements but are still made from dense materials.

25. D: It is an acceptable practice to sterilize an unpackaged extension cone paralleling (XCP) device when it will be used immediately following the sterilization cycle and can be transferred to the patient treatment area in a way that does not contaminate it with microbes. If this cannot be done, then it is not an acceptable practice to sterilize the item unpackaged and the dental team should have an alternative solution in place.

26. C: Radon is a colorless, odorless radioactive gas. It is produced by the decay of naturally occurring uranium in the soil. If a house is built on top of an area with high radon concentration, radon gas can seep into the house and accumulate. Radon exposure can go unnoticed for decades, but it is thought to be the second leading cause of lung cancer in the US. UV radiation is a specific wavelength of light rays, which represents minimal risk of harm. Cosmic radiation originates from outside of our planet, and fallout radiation is a by-product of nuclear detonations.

27. A: Chronic radiation exposure is something that could happen to dental staff members if they are not following protocol to keep themselves safe during patient radiation exposure. Chronic radiation exposure is being exposed to small amounts of radiation over a long period of time. This type of exposure has a long latent period; it is hard to link symptoms with a specific event because symptoms may not develop until 10 or 20 years after the chronic exposures.

28. A: Intraoral phosphor sensors are commonly found in dentistry alongside wired or direct digital sensors. Phosphor sensors must be covered with barriers before being placed in the mouth. They do not have antimicrobial properties that can decrease cross contamination, nor does the phosphor sensor processing machine have any disinfection capabilities. Phosphor sensors are removed from the mouth by the dental radiographer and must be removed with gloved hands because they will have saliva and microbes on them from the patient's oral cavity.

29. C: A floor is an example of a housekeeping surface. These surfaces have a low risk of disease transmission due to their location and minimal direct patient contact. They do not need to be cleaned between patients because they pose little risk and can be processed with less rigorous cleaners compared to other types of surfaces. These surfaces are generally cleaned on a routine basis, such as at the end of each day.

30. C: The maximum permissible dose (MPD) of radiation, which is set by the National Council on Radiation Protection and Measurements, states that the maximum permissible dose of occupational exposure to radiation is 5 rem. This limitation is set in order to protect workers from the dangerous effects of radiation exposure.

31. C: The hamulus is a piece of bone that extends outward from the area behind the last-erupted tooth in the upper arch. It cannot be felt with the tongue and does not stick out of the soft tissue, but it can be viewed on dental images; therefore, the dental radiographer should be familiar with it so it can be discussed with the patient if needed.

32. C: Several safeguards are in place to protect the operator from radiation exposure. The ALARA ("as low as reasonably achievable") principle applies to the operator as well. The operator's goal for radiation exposure should also be zero. The operator should refrain from standing in the line of the x-ray beam at any time. When pressing the exposure button, the operator should be at least 6 feet away or behind an appropriate barrier, such as drywall that is the appropriate thickness for blocking radiation. The operator needs to wear a dosimeter at all times while in the dental office to monitor exposure. Additionally, the dental office needs to maintain equipment appropriately to minimize exposure of everyone.

33. B: The density of a dental image is directly associated with the milliamp (mA) setting. The mA settings can be adjusted manually in older radiography machines and control how many electrons are created at the tungsten filament. Manufacturers of newer radiographic units allow for both the mA and kilovolt peak (kVp) to be increased or decreased at the same time, usually changed with the type of tooth being radiographed, if desired.

34. D: The federal requirement regarding the thickness of the aluminum filter on an x-ray machine operating at 70 kVp or greater is that the thickness of the aluminum filtration must be 2.5 mm. This thickness ensures that the long, low-energy wavelengths created, in addition to the useful wavelengths, are properly filtered and absorbed by the aluminum disks to prevent their emission.

35. C: Dental radiographers and other dental professionals must consider current injuries and infections that involve their hands when evaluating the appropriateness of providing patient care. When open lesions are present on the hands, the dental professional must remove themselves from all direct patient care and from handling patient care equipment until the condition has resolved.

36. B: Cone beam computed tomography (CBCT) allows for the ability to distinguish between the types of soft tissues present, which traditional dental panoramic imagery cannot. As in panoramic imagery, the ability to see impacted wisdom teeth, anomalies within the arches, and the view of the skull can also be seen in the CBCT radiograph.

37. A: Radiopaque areas on a dental image stand out as white areas or areas that are lighter in color. Areas appear white or light on an image when x-rays interact with an object and are unable to pass through it and strike the image receptor. This occurs with dense and thick objects. When x-rays strike these objects, they become lodged and interact with the object versus the sensor on the far side of the object. This can include the many shades of gray that can result with optimal dental tubehead settings. Radiolucent areas are darker and include structures such as gum tissue and the periodontal ligament: x-rays easily pass through these structures, allowing them to reach the image receptor and produce the pixels that form the dental image. Low-density and low-contrast areas will appear as darker areas on an image.

38. D: When the dental team is looking to diagnose mesial decay on tooth #29, the premolar bitewing would be the correct image to choose. This image will show the mesial area with the most clarity for the dental team, as well as demonstrate the most accurate angles.

39. C: Foreshortening is an exposure error that occurs when too many vertical angulations were used when the dental auxiliary was exposing the image receptor. The teeth will appear short and squat, possibly leading to improper tooth measurements during root canal therapy. To correct foreshortening, the dental auxiliary needs to decrease the amount of vertical angulation used.

40. C: The paralleling technique is used to reduce radiation exposure to the eye. With proper placement of the receptor parallel to the long axis of the tooth, the direction of the x-ray beam is directed specifically at the tooth to be radiographed rather than the eye. When proper techniques and receptor-holding devices are not used when taking dental radiographs, the risk for the eye to come in contact with the primary beam emitted is great.

41. B: It is still important to maintain safety even if a pediatric patient is uncooperative. The operator should not risk radiation exposure to stand in the line of the x-ray beam for any reason, including holding the sensors in place during x-rays. The best option would be to have the parent come and hold the child on their lap. Both the parent and child can be covered with the patient apron. If necessary, the parent can hold the sensor in place because this would be a single radiation exposure for the parent. Conversely, if the operator held the sensor, this would risk repeated exposures, which may lead to adverse health effects in the future.

42. D: Due to the dangers of excess secondary or scatter radiation, it has been determined that the dental auxiliary should be concerned if their weekly dose of radiation exceeds 100 milliroentgens (mR). A dosage above this level could put the dental auxiliary at unnecessary occupational risk for the effects of radiation exposure.

43. C: The dental team should be trained on and be aware of the maximum permissible dose (MPD). This is a standard and a benchmark that identifies the highest amount of radiation that someone can be exposed to without interventions needing to occur. This will be measured within a specific time frame. There are basic recommendations that the dental team should study and review during team meetings. This knowledge should be paired with the use of radiation monitoring badges that are monitored and documented for employee records.

44. A: The use of a biological indicator and the processing of this item is the only way that the dental team can identify if sterilization has actually occurred for a given instrument load. These biological indicators come in different forms, but all of them will contain live microbes that are harmless and are used to assess if the sterilization machine kills the microbes during its standard cycle. Following use of a biological indicator in an instrument load, the dental team can process it in house or send it to a lab for testing. If there are still live microbes found, that means that sterilization did not occur. If all pathogens have been killed during the load, sterilization has been achieved. Physical and chemical indicators are helpful in assessing that the sterilization machine has reached the proper time, temperature, and pressure, but not that it actually killed all living microbes in a given instrument load.

45. C: An XCP device is an example of a semicritical instrument used in dental imaging. Semicritical instruments include sensor holders (e.g., the Snap-A-Ray device) as well as beam alignment devices. These items are placed into the oral cavity and come into contact with tissues inside the mouth but do not pass through these tissues.

46. A: The patient apron is an optional protective mechanism that can be used in dentistry; due to how it is used, it is classified as a noncritical instrument or item. This means that it is associated with a very low risk of disease transmission. This classification also allows for chemicals and disinfectants that are of lower strength to be used to clean and disinfect it. This is an item that only comes into contact with the patient and operator's skin and clothing; therefore, less rigorous disinfection is needed.

47. B: When performing infection control practices with PSPs, the dental radiographer must always wear gloves because the PSPs will have been in contact with the patient's saliva and oral fluids. PSPs are required to be placed into barriers before they are used because they cannot withstand heat sterilization nor immersion sterilization methods.

48. B: When a patient needs to have bitewing images taken in a partially edentulous area, cotton rolls can be placed in the area to substitute the missing teeth. When the patient closes on the bitewing tab, their teeth, along with the cotton rolls, will stabilize the tab while the image is being taken.

49. D: A properly exposed bitewing will not show periapical radiolucent pathology because the apices of the teeth are not seen in a bitewing x-ray. The crestal bone, interproximal areas between the teeth, and images of the maxillary and mandibular crowns should all be seen in a diagnostically acceptable bitewing radiograph.

50. C: It is important for the dental auxiliary to stabilize any image receptor holding device that is used during the placement of image receptors in the patient's mouth. If this is not done, the image receptor may slip, resulting in a crooked or slanted picture. This may result in a retake if the dentist is not able to view pathological conditions or areas in question.

51. D: Movement of the patient during panoramic exposure will result in blurred imagery. The blurred structure will be found in the area in which the patient actually moved, or the cassette came in contact with the patient's shoulders due to faulty positioning of the patient prior to exposure. Just as in regular photography, movement can often cause distortion.

52. C: Nerve tissue is the least likely of the cell groups of tissue to be affected by exposure to dental radiation. This is due to the fact that nerves are located deep within muscle tissue or bone, such as the skull. Although nerve tissue is abundant in the human body, it is also usually located beneath the protective layers of tissues or bone.

53. B: When alcohol-based hand rubs are used, the dental team must rub their hands together until they are dry and the product has been absorbed into the skin. This is a product that should only be used when hands are relatively clean; it should not be used with soap and water, but as a replacement for them. When used properly, alcohol-based hand rubs are very effective at killing microbes on hands, which has resulted in this product being widely used in dentistry today. The optimal amount of alcohol in products for dentistry averages approximately 70%.

54. A: While there are many ways to achieve infection control in dental radiology, applying plastic barriers over image receptors is the best way to prevent cross-contamination. These plastic barriers prevent the image receptors from coming into contact with the patient's oral tissues and saliva, which reduces the chance of cross-contamination.

55. B: The safest place for the dental auxiliary to stand during radiation exposure to a patient would be at a right angle, or 90-135 degrees to the source of radiation or the tubehead. Standing at this angle will prevent any secondary or scatter radiation that may have been generated by the primary beam interacting with the patient.

56. B: Digital radiography is very advantageous to dental offices but it also has disadvantages. Losing the receptors is usually not a disadvantage for digital radiography as long as the digital images are appropriately backed up. Cost can be a disadvantage because purchasing the setup equipment can be costly. Training employees to use the equipment as well as the software can be a disadvantage. Infection control can also be an issue because the sensor or PSP plates are not able to be heat sanitized. These items must have a protective barrier when used with a patient and must be carefully cleaned according to manufacturer's instructions.

57. D: When capturing dental images, the dental team should always place the image receptor parallel to the teeth or the structures being radiographed. The receptor and the tooth are then in the same plane or the same landscape, which will allow for the structure to be captured with accurate dimensions. If the receptor was placed perpendicular to the structure being captured, this would result in a right angle and the structure would be pushed onto the receptor at this angle, resulting in a large amount of distortion and a lack of ability to diagnose pathological conditions, including dental decay.

58. A: Federal requirements are in place to control the types of x-rays that are released from an x-ray machine. The aluminum filter captures long wavelengths before they leave the x-ray tube. Long wavelengths are harmful to the patient and operator and are not needed to produce dental x-rays. Federal regulations state that all x-ray machines using 70 kVp or more must use an aluminum filter measuring 2.5 mm. The lead collimator also helps to control radiation exposure by controlling the size and shape of the x-ray beam. Rectangular-shaped beams reduce the amount of radiation exposure. The position-indicating device (PID) is available in 2 sizes: short and long. The long size measuring 12-16 inches tends to reduce the amount of radiation exposure because the beam does not spread as much as the shorter size.

59. D: Digital radiography is becoming very popular in dentistry for many reasons. One important reason is that using digital technologies and image receptors decrease the amount of radiation that needs to be used by 50% to 90%, depending on the type of imaging system used. This, along with the ease of viewing dental images and the speed with which the dentist has access to these images, are all reasons why many dental offices are choosing to make the switch to digital technologies.

60. C: The retromolar pad is the area that is found distal to the last erupted tooth on the mandibular arch, therefore, it will be found in the mandibular molar periapical.

61. A: When performing patient care in the dental office, including imaging techniques, the dental radiographer and other dental staff can perform hand hygiene in a number of ways including washing with soap and water, using antimicrobial soap, using alcohol-based hand rubs, and wearing surgical scrubs when required. The technique used is dependent on the patient and the procedure, which the dental radiographer must be familiar with. Transient flora refers to the bacteria that naturally exist on human skin and within the human body; they are not harmful or capable of causing infection. These are also the type of bacteria that can easily be removed when hands are cleaned appropriately.

62. B: The type of radiation that is created when the primary beam comes in contact with any matter is called "secondary radiation." An example: Secondary radiation is formed when the primary radiation comes in contact with the patient's skin during exposure.

63. D: There are many advantages to digital radiography in dental offices. Photostimulable storage phosphor (PSP) plates are often used to assist with imaging. The images must first be processed using a processing device that scans the images. PSP plates expose the patient to less radiation and they are thinner and more comfortable for the patient than other types of sensors. Digital radiography allows for instant communication with other dentists or dental professionals if needed for consultation. Digital radiography allows for manipulation of the image as needed for more or less contrast, enlargement of the image, or placement of different colors for diagnostic or viewing purposes.

64. B: Elongation is an exposure error that occurs when too few vertical angulations are used; this is the opposite of foreshortening. Any time that elongation occurs, the dental auxiliary needs to increase the vertical angulations. This will correct the error and result in the structures appearing in their realistic dimensions.

65. D: When using the paralleling technique during periapical exposure, the sensor and the long axis of the tooth are parallel to each other; otherwise, distortion will result. At no time will the sensor and the long axis of the tooth be perpendicular to each other. During the bisecting angle technique, the long axis of the tooth is established and the sensor is placed at a right angle to an imaginary bisecting line that divides the angle created by the long axis and the imaginary line.

66. D: The ALARA concept reminds us that the patient's exposure to dental radiation should be maintained to a degree of "as low as reasonably achievable." This concept is encouraged to be practiced by dental staff; it is a constant reminder that if a dental x-ray is needed, it should be obtained at the very first attempt. Time and proper technique are needed to follow this concept before the exposure is given.

67. C: When a pregnant patient presents at the dental office, there should be no deviation from the standard care of practice that would be used on a nonpregnant patient. Due to the low doses of radiation used in dentistry, the previous recommendations to avoid dental exposure during pregnancy have been revoked.

68. D: The term "frequency" can be defined as the number of wavelengths that pass a given point in a certain specified time period. A wavelength can be defined as the distance between two crests of a wave. The shorter the wavelength, the faster the frequency of the wave, and the longer the wavelength, the slower the frequency of the wave. Velocity can be defined as the speed of a wave.

69. B: When the dental auxiliary is exposing an occlusal radiograph, a size 4 image receptor should be used in order to capture adequate areas of the arch being radiographed. If a smaller size were used, important parts of the image may be cut off of the resulting image.

70. A: The inverted Y is a formation that is created by the walls of the maxillary sinus and the wall of the nasal cavity coming together. When these two bony areas meet, it causes an upside-down Y area to appear, known as the inverted Y. This image may appear in the center of a maxillary canine periapical.

71. A: Reproductive cells are the group of cells that are most likely to be affected by radiation. If radiation is able to penetrate the reproductive cell on a molecular level, the radiation may be able to alter the deoxyribonucleic acid (DNA) structure of such cells. Often, this disruption of the DNA forces the cell to not survive or the DNA mutates into abnormal DNA. Because the normal reproductive cell is composed primarily of water, oftentimes the DNA is not affected, but the water molecular bonds are. These bonds, once broken, can cause toxins to form, which ultimately can kill the cell.

72. C: An extracted tooth needs to be treated as if it is potentially infectious. They are considered regulated waste and should be disposed of in a medical waste bag. Regulated waste needs to be properly labeled, packaged, and transported to a medical waste facility. Special containers are used that are hard and leak proof, and can withstand transport without breaking. Most dental offices will contract with a company that specializes in removal of regulated waste. If the extracted tooth is to be saved for the patient or for use in education, it must be sterilized first. Heat sterilization can be used if amalgam is not present in the tooth. A tooth that contains amalgam cannot be heat sterilized because of the potential for mercury vapors to result. In this case, the tooth can be soaked in glutaraldehyde for 30 minutes to disinfect.

73. A: A dark shadow obscuring the apices of the maxillary teeth will be seen on a panoramic image when the patient's tongue is not kept at the roof of the mouth during exposure. Improper placement of the tongue will not impair the diagnostic value of what is seen on the mandibular teeth.

74. A: A dental assistant is considered an occupationally exposed individual to radiation. It is important to monitor exposure to radiation over the long term. There are 2 ways to measure exposure. The traditional system uses roentgen (R), the radiation absorbed dose (rad), and the roentgen equivalent in man (rem). The other system is newer and utilizes the metric system. It is called the International System of Units (SI). It measures radiation using coulomb per kilogram (c/kg), the gray (Gy), and the sievert (Sv). The National Council on Radiation Protection and Measurements (NCRP) sets the standard for the Maximum Permissible Dose (MPD). For the general public, the MPD is 0.1 rem/year (or 0.001 Sv/year using the SI system). For pregnant employees with occupational exposure, it is 0.5 rem/year (or 0.005 Sv/year using the SI system). For other workers with occupational exposure, it is 5 rem/year (0.05 Sv/year using SI system). The cumulative lifetime dose is calculated by multiplying 10 mSv times the age of the employee in years.

75. A: The definition of the Frankfort plane, as used in dental radiography, is a plane that passes through the floor of the orbit and to the external auditory meatus. This imaginary line is a point of reference that can be used to assist in the placement or positioning of the patient's head, prior to dental radiographic exposure. This plane should remain parallel to the floor for optimal results.

76. D: When exposing a premolar or bicuspid image, if the distal of the cuspid or canine is not on the image receptor, the dental auxiliary needs to move the image receptor more anterior in the mouth in order to capture this structure. It is important for the dentist to have an adequate view of the distal of the canine in order to diagnose any pathology that may be occurring in this area.

77. B: The coronoid process is a mandibular anatomical structure but appears in the maxillary molar periapical image. This is due to how the image receptor is placed in the mouth and the angulations used when capturing this image. The mental foramen will appear in the mandibular premolar image, the genial tubercles will appear in the mandibular central periapical, and the tuberosity will appear in the maxillary molar periapical image.

78. A: In the field of dentistry, high doses of radiation cannot be produced by the standard dental tubehead. Even when the settings on the control panel are increased, it is still not possible to produce extreme amounts of radiation resulting in acute exposures. This would occur in situations such as nuclear power plant leaks, or radiation therapy for cancer treatment.

79. C: When using the paralleling technique during intraoral periapical exposure, the receptor should be placed as far away as possible from the lingual surface of the teeth, near the middle of the mouth. This ensures that the patient will be placed in such a way that the long axis of the tooth will be parallel to the placement of the receptor.

80. D: When the dentist requires a periapical image, it is to view the complete structure of the teeth being imaged. This includes everything from the apex or tip of the root all the way to the crown of the teeth. The placement of the receptor for periapical images allows for structures to appear on the image with the correct anatomical dimensions. Occlusal images are used to see structures in three dimensions. Bitewing images are used to capture the crowns of the teeth and are the tool used to detect interproximal dental decay on the teeth.

It's Your Moment, Let's Celebrate It!

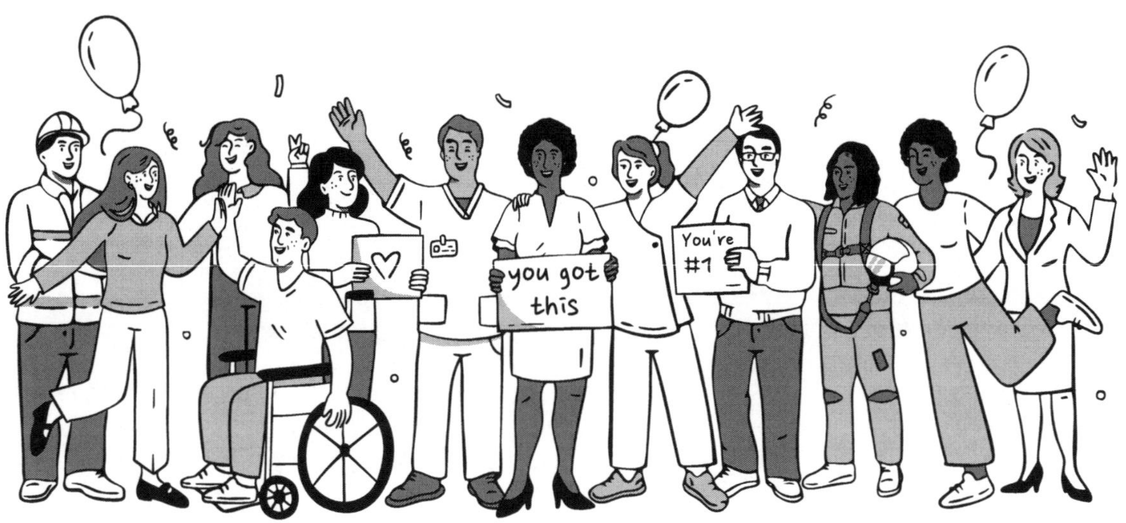

Share your story @mometrixtestpreparation